THE BAD FOOD MYTH

lose weight by learning to love yourself

Tracy Hancock

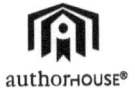

authorHOUSE®

AuthorHouse™ UK Ltd.
500 Avebury Boulevard
Central Milton Keynes, MK9 2BE
www.authorhouse.co.uk
Phone: 08001974150

First published by AuthorHouse 4/8/2010

ISBN: 978-1-4490-8041-9 (sc)

This book is printed on acid-free paper.

Acknowledgements

I would like to thank my sister Julie, my dad Terry
and stepmum Pauline
for all their love, support and encouragement.

My friends Leesa and Sarah for taking the time
to read my book and give me feedback.

My husband Peter for making this possible.

And finally Marc for all his hard work and for
putting my book to the test to prove it works.

Thank you everyone.

Dedications

To my husband Peter whom I love more than
anything.
And in loving memory of my mum
Pauline Nugent 'a very special lady.'

Introduction

Have you ever wondered why it is that whilst there are literally hundreds of 'diets' to choose from, some new, some of which have been around for years, all 'guaranteeing' that 'amazing new you', yet as a population, we are actually getting fatter and becoming less healthy.

I certainly have, which is why I felt compelled to write this book.

For many years people, including myself, have known that by and large 'diets' don't work, some people lose their weight by starving themselves, some people even resort to making themselves sick but in most instances the vast majority of 'dieters' only end up putting all the weight back on, sometimes with a little extra thrown in. Most people on a diet will also tell you they are miserable and unhappy with themselves, never seeming to achieve that 'ideal' weight which they believe will bring them happiness.

Trying to look like *that* model we've see in *this* magazine just feeds into our emotional insecurities and leads us back to food for comfort. In fact you can put your scales away because you won't need them. We know within ourselves how we feel, and whether or not we are eating a balanced diet, the hard part is acting upon what we know and hopefully this is where I can help.

I know what you are thinking; "so what's new, what are you going to tell me that's any different to what's been said before?" My answer 'everything' because my book is not a diet book and you will not be counting calories, yet you will lose weight. How you may ask, well through learning to love and nurture yourself by finding out what it is you actually need to comfort yourself instead of food.

My book will take you on a journey that will explore your relationship with food, where it comes from and how to change it. This will be done through various exercises that get you to look into yourself to find out what happens for you emotionally when you eat so as to establish what 'void' you may be trying to fill with food. By doing this you will begin to understand your eating habits and be able to make an 'informed' choice to fill this void with what you really need.

My book will give you insight into where your eating 'struggle' stems from, and how you can begin to do things differently. I will *not* be encouraging you to lose weight that will happen naturally once you understand your relationship with food and can make different choices.

You will be empowered to free yourself from the 'emotion – void – food' cycle while also learning that food in itself is not bad it is how you choose to use the food, hence the book title 'The Bad Food Myth'.

A word of warning, looking into yourself emotionally is not easy. Having had my own psychotherapy for more than five years I speak from my own experiences, some good, some not so good, but the rewards are life changing because they begin the process of enabling us to start loving and nurturing ourselves.

Once we start to love ourselves for who we are we can let go of pursuing that unattainable 'perfect' figure, and really start to appreciate what we have. The result is you lose weight without ever needing to diet because you no longer need to use food as an emotional crutch.

So if you feel you are ready to challenge yourself emotionally and are prepared to be totally honest with yourself, while taking responsibility for *your* choices in life, knowing that even though some choices are difficult, *you* can choose something different, this is the book for you.

The reward will be that you start to understand why you comfort eat and what 'void' you are trying to fill with food and you will begin to fill it with something much better, while at the same time loosing weight and liking yourself a lot more along the way.

Finally before you begin your journey it is important to mention that some of you will have deep emotional needs that this book cannot deal with; if this is the case and you feel you want to deal with these issues appropriately you may look to engage in your own therapy.

Chapter 1

Only you can change your life

It is important to understand that although I can guide and advise you the emphasis has to be on *you* as an individual because there is only you who can change your life by making different choices. Everyone is unique, meaning there is no 'one way fits all' solution. We all have to decide what will work in our lives and what changes we are prepared to make.

Since we are all unique individuals, what works for one person in terms of eating and lifestyle may not work for someone else, which is just one of the reasons, amongst others, that diets don't work. We are not 'designed' to fit into someone else's idea of what works.

Literally hundreds of diet books have been written, telling us what we should eat, and how, if we follow their regime, we can change our lives. The problem with these regimes is that they are not practical or realistic. They are written by people who do not live the average 9-5 lifestyle, so although the theory may be sound the practicalities are very hard to maintain in 'real life'.

Only *you* know what's 'livable' for you, and what you can realistically cope with in terms of a lifestyle change, because only *you* will know what void you are trying to fill through food.

Food is often about much more than being hungry

If we only ate when we were hungry being overweight would not be the concern it is, providing of course we ate sensibly. The truth is food is 'attached' to so many emotional issues very few people, if any, actually eat only when they are hungry. We all eat for numerous different reasons, hunger being only one. This is fine, providing it's balanced eating, it is only when the balance is missing that things become a problem.

Too much food and we become overweight, too little food and we become underweight both of which can cause emotional and physical problems.

Food will *never* fill an emotional void, which is why at times we can eat, and eat, and eat and never feel full. *Food will only ever fill our biological hunger.* Sure, it may make you feel good for a little while but if you are eating to try and fill an emotional need you will only end up feeling worse.

Physiologically when you have eaten, especially sweet foods your body gets a sugar rush and this creates a false high so you automatically feel better but the problem is this high does not last. As your blood sugar drops so will the false high created by the food, so if you have eaten to feel better or to comfort yourself you will feel worse and more importantly your emotional need is still unmet.

Most people will have some issues with food

Most people will have some issues that come out via food. It is not just people who are overweight / underweight, or those whose health is affected, but these are the people society often focuses upon because of the 'visual' aspect, in that we can *see* their problem, whereas with other people we may not be able to.

Bulimics, for example, have many psychological issues that present through food, often because food is the only thing they feel they can have control over. Bulimics will also usually have health issues, often serious, but they can habitually hide it better because 'visually, they look 'normal'. The whole process of binge eating and then 'purging', physically making themselves sick, allows the body just enough time to begin digesting some of the food they've eaten, which means they often maintain a visually healthy weight, so other people often never realize what's going on.

Anorexics too have severe emotional issues that come out via food but again with the way society is in terms of image people condone being extremely thin and are often praising this type of figure, rather than seeing it for what it is; 'unhealthy'. I am not suggesting everyone who is thin is anorexic, but I do believe many very thin people also have issues with food even if they are not anorexic.

The human body was not designed to be 'stick' thin. Generally woman after puberty carry around 30% more body fat than men, to enable them to have children. So why are most women so desperate to get rid of this healthy natural fat that their body needs - to fit into some stereotype of what so called beauty is. I find this very sad.

Everyone has a relationship with food

Overweight or underweight, we know ourselves whether or not our relationship with food is affecting our life; we don't really need someone else to confirm it. What we do need to do is acknowledge this, as this will enable us to do something about it and find out what the underlying emotional issue/s are. Our relationship with food will often have developed in our childhood, as a result of how we interpreted, and made sense of what food meant for our family and us.

We will *always* have a relationship with food because it is such an important part of our lives, but if we can make sense of this relationship, and determine whether it is unhealthy or healthy, we can begin to make food work for us rather than against us.

Ultimately we cannot survive without food, unlike other things we may have an unhealthy relationship with i.e. drink, drugs, gambling, overspending, etc. that we can live without, food we cannot. If we stopped eating we would eventually die!

Therefore our relationship with food becomes far more complex and often ends up being a love hate relationship; it may at times feel like food has some kind of control over us, when the reality is *WE* HAVE

THE CONTROL, FOOD CANNOT CONTROL US UNLESS WE LET IT BECAUSE IT IS AN INANIMATE OBJECT.

The challenge

So this is the challenge: For *you* to take responsibility for your life and stop ignoring the power you have within you to do something different. If you continue to dismiss this power nothing will change, and this won't be just in terms of food.

Regrettably, this 'pattern' of not taking responsibility has a tendency to filter through into other aspects of our lives, and has in fact, in many ways, become part of our society. Leading to a 'blame culture', where people begin to think everything that happens to them *must* be someone or something else's fault. Unfortunately when this happens we end up being left with very little control over anything in our lives.

This *is* a very big challenge, and not one that happens overnight. It is a life choice, but a choice you *are* capable of making. No one said life would always be easy but it can become easier if you let it. The alternative is to continue to believe it's everyone else's fault but then you will never achieve what you want because you are waiting for someone or something else to change things for you rather than realizing *you can do it yourself.*

For instance, people continually blame fast food restaurants, the government, supermarkets etc for the obesity crisis rather than looking within themselves. Obviously the rise of fast foods chains, processed foods and addictive foods has not helped *but* and this is a big but you still have a choice whether you choose to eat this type of food. No one forces you to.

I am not suggesting the choice is easy but how great to realize we can choose, food does not have to control us we can in fact control it. Food is only our enemy if we let it be. No one food is either 'bad' or 'good' hence the 'bad food myth'. It is you who makes the food bad or good depending on how you choose to use it.

Example

Most people would argue that vegetables are 'good' foods full of healthy vitamins and nutrients and while this is true if this was all you were choosing to eat your body would be undernourished. In the same way chips are seen as a 'bad' food with very little nutritional benefit but if you chose to eat them only occasionally what harm would that do in terms of your health; very little.

You can now begin to see that it is what you decide to do with food that makes it healthy or unhealthy. Anything in moderation is fine and if you can really get to grips with this concept it is truly liberating because you literally can eat anything you want as long as you stick to the principal of 'everything in moderation'.

As adults we need to accept the fact that *we* have choices, and it is down to *us* how we use them, we must stop blaming others for what is ultimately *our* decision. There is always a choice, which at times may not be the easiest one, but a choice nevertheless.

Love yourself

Having an unhealthy relationship with food shows a lack of love for you. You deserve to treat your body better, and you are worth taking care of. You need to ask yourself why you don't think enough of yourself to look after you and your body properly? You need to begin to love the body you have and the individual within it and then I truly believe you will begin to take better care of yourself and your relationship with food *will* change for the better.

When your relationship to yourself and food changes you should never need to diet again, because your lifestyle will change and you will want to look after yourself. You can then begin to love the person you are and the body you have.

You can let go of your unhealthy relationship with food by understanding what it is about, which will enable you to can get your needs met in a more productive and beneficial way. Once you do your body should begin to find its own natural weight. It just needs to be given the chance and then you will begin to eat more when you are hungry and less for an emotional need.

You can still enjoy food

You can still enjoy food, I do, but I now know when enough is enough, and I know sufficient about myself to realize when I am eating because of an emotional need. This doesn't mean I never do it, but what it does mean is I am aware that it is not actually about my being hungry, and I begin to think about what I really need at this point.

Example

I may be feeling particularly low one day and fancy a cream cake or crisps, so I let myself have them. I do not deprive myself, but I also recognize that there may be something else going on. I ask myself 'what is it that I need at this moment to stop me turning to food for comfort and what am I really craving'?

By doing this I retain the control, I do not let the food control me. It also means I am able to get what I may need at this vulnerable time while keeping my relationship with food 'ok'. So I do not go into feeling even worse because I ate a cream cake or crisps and it also means I do not make food bad or good.

Everything is about balance and as long as the balance stays roughly central you shouldn't have a problem. It's when the balance starts to shift off centre that things may go wrong, that's when your warning bells need to be going off, so you can quickly do what is necessary to re-address the balance before it gets out of control.

Chapter 2

As Adults we get to choose

As children our choices are limited because our parents need to hold ultimate responsibility for us. They make the majority of decisions because we are not mature enough emotionally or physically. Unfortunately sometimes these decisions are not actually what is right for us at that time and we can experience them as damaging.

We need to remember that for the most part parents believe they are acting in their child's best interests, however because adults and children think differently what a parent thinks is appropriate does not necessarily match up with what the child thinks, even when the adults decision is made from a well meaning place.

Example

When I was a child my parents decided I needed to move school because they felt the school I was at would not give me as good an education. They believed by moving me I would have a better start in life and have wider access to future opportunities such as university and employment.

Obviously as an adult this thought process totally makes sense but to a young child who does not think logically or rationally all I saw was me being forcibly moved from all my friends to a school where I did not know anyone and did not want to be. I felt my parents were being cruel and uncaring when actually for them it was the opposite; their decision came from the fact they did care and obviously weren't aware of or hadn't considered the potential negative outcomes of such a move.

I therefore experienced this decision as damaging to me because as a child I did not understand the adult reasons for the move.

Every child will have experienced incidents like this in their past because no one has 'perfect' parents. These events are difficult and will undoubtedly have affected you, and 'shaped' the person you have become. What is important to remember is as adults we have choices available to us that we did not have as children.

We now control our own lives and are therefore responsible for how they turn out; we cannot as adults blame other people because we are no longer children who *need* to be dependent.

You have to want to change

Once we are adults we need to become responsible for ourselves and understand that we now have choices and can make our own decisions.

Only *you* can decide how you want the rest of your life to be, and how *you* want to be. At the end of the day it is you who must decide to make changes no one else can do this for you.

One of the most important things I've learned as a Psychotherapist is that we cannot help people unless they are willing to help themselves, and they must be prepared to do something different. Yes we can 'facilitate', by making people aware of their processes, behaviours and patterns, and where they may have originated. We can give people options to be different, but that person still has to choose to do something different, and be ready to do so. *They have to want it for themselves.*

You will already know this if you've ever tried to give up something for someone else, when *you* weren't ready to. I'm fairly confident that eventually, not only will you have failed, the chances are you either ended up resenting the person that 'made' you do it, or you beat yourself up for not being able to stick with it.

However, if you've ever given something up because you really wanted to, and *you* were ready to, you will probably have succeeded, because it was *your* decision.

Example

For example when a father tells his daughter not to see her boyfriend because he believes him to be 'no good' what normally happens is the daughter will continue to see her boyfriend but behind her father's back because she is not ready to finish it. Once she realizes for herself that he is 'no good' and feels ready she will usually finish with him without any encouragement.

Whatever you decide is fine

So you may read this book and decide you're not ready to do something different, *that's fine* you are an adult and it's *your* choice. You can always come back to it if, or when, you feel you are ready. Equally you may read this book and want to continue ignoring your relationship with food because that's easier for you and *that's all right too* again it's your decision.

You may read this and think you are ready, but then not be able to put in place the things needed to achieve what you want, *again that's fine.* A few may read this and it may enable them to change their lives, and their relationship with food because they were ready, *which is great.*

Whatever you do you are still 'ok'. Having an unhealthy relationship with food does not define *you* as a person, even though you may feel it does, especially if your health is affected. You are still a good person, the eating is a 'behaviour' that *can* be changed or altered, the core of you is still you and you are *amazing.*

If only one person reads this book and feels better, or begins to deal with their relationship with food then that's great, because this is *not* a book about slimming or trying to lose weight. This book is about getting to understand why we eat the way we do. What we may actually need instead of food. How we might obtain this and most importantly how we start loving ourselves more.

We also have to accept that we all have different bodies,

just as we are all individuals. Difference is good and healthy. It only becomes unhealthy when we try to make our bodies into something they are not designed to be, like trying to become a size zero even if this means eating next to nothing and putting our health at risk.

Accepting responsibility gives us the power to change

The belief that food is bad is a myth because food alone is not bad, yes certain foods may be detrimental to our health if eaten to excess, but again, if eaten in balance they are not. *We* make food bad in our choice of how to use it, how we eat it, and how often we eat it.

Example

If you choose to eat fast food once a month this would not be considered unhealthy but if you choose to eat fast food every night this would be. Yet it is you that chooses whether or not to eat the fast food daily or monthly meaning it is you who makes the food unhealthy. The same way as a seemingly healthy food like salad would be unhealthy for you if it was all you chose to eat because it would not have all the essential vitamins and minerals your body needs.

I'm sure you will have heard all the usual arguments (perhaps even used them on occasion) such as: "but the problem is, there are more fast food restaurants than ever" or "everywhere you go there's 'junk' food". Once more we're looking to 'blame' someone or something else. *We have a choice, we're adults.*

When was the last time that you heard of someone having been kidnapped, and then being forced to eat in a fast food restaurant?

We *choose* to go into them and *we* choose what we eat once we're in there. Fast food restaurants, don't make us unhealthy, *our choices do.* If nobody went to these restaurants they would go out of business, instead there's an abundance of them, and by choosing to go in *we* are keeping them in business, nothing else.

If you have a take away or junk food once a month, or even once a week, but are eating a varied balanced diet the rest of the time, this will not make you unhealthy, or overweight. It is only when the balance tips in favour of fast/junk food as the *main* food of choice, that you make it become unhealthy.

Balance is the key, if the balance is affected ask yourself why? What is going on for me at this moment that means I need to eat more, or get comfort from food? What am I avoiding, or trying to fill, what might I need instead?

Chapter 3

Are you addicted to food?

As I said in the introduction this book is not going to give you all the answers or suddenly make you thin, this book is about embracing *you* as a person, for who *you* are and how *your* body was meant to be, not you trying to fit into an image that society 'demands'.

With that said let's go!

(You will need a pen and some paper)

Begin to think about the following questions, write down your answers or thoughts as you go. Your answers to the questions are intended to give you a sense of what 'emotions' you linked to food when you were a child, and to try and give you an understanding of what's going on now and where those 'emotions' stem from.

Questions:

What do you remember about your childhood in relation to food?

What meals did you eat?

Where did you eat them?

Who cooked?

What do you remember about meal times?

Who ate what in your family, was anyone 'fussy'?

What kind of figures did your immediate family have, mum, dad, grandma, granddad, brothers, sisters, etc?

What appetites did they have, who liked their food, who didn't?

What food did you like, dislike?

Could you decide what you ate, if not, who decided?

Who decided what time you ate?

Could you leave food when you were full, if not what happened?

Were certain foods used as rewards for good behaviours?

If you showed emotion did food become involved i.e. if you were crying were you given something to eat, sweets etc?

At school what went on around meals, what choices did you have?

Did you eat school dinners or a packed lunch?

If packed lunch, who chose what went into it and what you ate?

Can you remember any messages around food and eating i.e. waste not want not etc?

Do you know anything about your appetite as a baby, how you were fed, were you underweight, overweight, etc?

What does food mean to you now, can you take it or leave it or does your life revolve around it? Do you live to eat or eat to live?

Now try to remember any 'memories' you have associated with food, good or bad, and write them down as well.

Food as a positive experience.

Eating is commonly a very 'social' occasion, and can be a time when families sit down collectively and spend time together, perhaps recalling what has gone on for them that day. This can make people feel happy because they are getting contact and recognition, which we all need.

However, what *can* happen is we begin to believe that it is actually the food that is making us feel good, and not the contact and recognition, so whenever we feel down, sad, lonely, etc. throughout our lives we look to food as a means of recapturing those feelings of happiness we had as children.

Sometimes in our childhood food has been used purposely to make us feel better such as when we hurt ourselves, or when we may have been sad. While this is not a bad thing to do it can mean that later in life when we are adults we use this same method of coping to comfort ourselves when things go wrong or are difficult.

What we fail to realize is that it wasn't actually the food that created those happy feelings, and though I'm not saying food isn't nice, it can create a false 'high'. What we need to recognize is that the being with other people is what made us feel good not the food, which is why no matter what, how much or how often we eat, our feelings and emotions very quickly return, and the struggle with food and emotions continues.

So how can you begin to get your emotional needs met, and get the appreciation, contact and attachment you need instead of looking in the fridge.

Food as a negative experience

For other people meal times may have been an 'empty' time emotionally, without any social contact, so for them the food began to fill their isolation and for a little while gave them some comfort from their being alone.

Unfortunately, before too long they turn to food for almost every emotional time in their lives. They begin to eat when they are sad, frightened, and angry, even eating when they are happy. These people rather than 'feeling' the emotions that they *need* to experience in their lives use food as a substitute for those emotions, because feeling emotions is often hard.

When we are children we need permission from our parents to have our feelings because this is how we learn feelings are ok. If for whatever reason our parents struggled with giving us this permission we often grow up believing it's not alright to express certain feelings.

Often when this happens and parents have failed to give their child the appropriate support they need when having their feelings, by the time we become adults we have little sense of knowing that it's alright to have feelings, and that we will get through them. This is usually when we turn to other things to try and manage our emotions, such as food. What you need to learn is how to comfort yourself, but not through food.

Summary

Food in some households may have been used in different ways:

As a reward,

As a punishment; or

As a way to stop you feeling your emotions.

For example:

How often have we seen a child cry only to hear someone say

"Come on don't cry, its okay, have a sweet"

Not realizing that the child will begin to associate sweets, or other treats, with making them feel better, and may then go on to try and do the same with food as an adult.

When a child does something wrong they may have been punished by being told;

"For that, you can go to your room without any tea"

By not being allowed their tea they begin to associate not having food with feeling bad, so having food *must* make you feel good.

Equally in some households food was used in celebrations, so if we achieved something good, or on birthdays, we got our favourite food. So here again the happy feeling becomes linked with the food rather than the achievement itself. We can then begin to believe it is actually the food that will make us feel good, and endeavour to recreate this when we are older.

It's important to remember that food will always be used in the ways I have mentioned and I am not suggesting otherwise. What we need is to start seeing food for what it is. Yes it is often enjoyable to eat, but if we can be conscious of what else is happening around us that may be affecting us emotionally, we can begin to see more clearly what is making us feel good. Maybe it's the company we're in, maybe it's our birthday, or maybe we have achieved something good in our lives.

We need to be aware that although many social situations do involve food it is unlikely to be the food on its own that enables us to have a positive experience. It is also worth noting that there are many other ways to celebrate and socialize that don't have to revolve around food.

The power of the mind

The subconscious is very powerful and what we need to realize is that a lot of our 'choices' are made unconsciously, without thinking, but the more we do think about them, the more we become aware of them, and the more we begin to understand them. Only then do we have the option to choose to do something different, and if we feel we are not yet ready to do something different, that's fine, but at least now we can understand some of our 'behaviour' in relation to food.

The key is to discover what you enjoy doing, and to look at how you might have a good time without food, if you do involve food, fine, just be aware that it may *not* be the food that is creating that 'feel good' factor.

Not convinced?

If you are still unsure about what I mean ask yourself these questions.

Have you ever eaten to feel better, if so what happened?

How long did the 'good' feeling last? (If you had one)

The likelihood is you're remembering that shortly after you ate you began feeling guilty or angry with yourself, and then you gave yourself a hard time, beginning the process of 'self-loathing'. Now you actually feel worse than you did before you ate, so the 'cycle' continues, unless, *you* choose to change the way in which you look to fill the 'void', and meet whatever 'need' you're missing in a different more healthy way.

From the day we are born until the day we die we often use food as if it were an emotional 'crutch'. Fortunately, by becoming aware of how and why we do this, we *can* choose if we want to do something differently, something that might actually make us feel better about ourselves afterwards, not worse. This process is not easy, if it were, *weight* would not be the issue it has become.

It all comes down to *your* choice of lifestyle, what *you* want to do and how *you* want to be, it's *your* life, no one said life would always be easy, and some of the choices you have to make will be difficult, but *you* will be in control, *you get to choose.*

Chapter 4

Exercise

(You will need your pen and paper)

Write down your earliest memory of food,

How old were you?

What do you remember about it?

Do you remember what it was?

What did it taste like?

How did it make you feel?

Who else was there, what were they doing?

Was it an occasion, if so what?

What day of the week was it, what time of day?

Did you eat a lot, a little, average?

Were you full?

Is your main memory the food or what was going on around you?

Try to become aware of how you are feeling now about this memory.

What is it bringing up for you?

How does this event relate to your eating now? (As an adult)

Has it influenced your eating in any way?

Was it the start of a pattern of eating in your life?

Did a pattern develop later on?

Really spend some time on this, think about what you are writing down and how you are feeling, how does it link to the present, if at all, can you relate it to the questions you answered earlier.

An example of my own.

One of my first memories of food is having Sunday dinner. I believe the reason I remember this more than other times is because it was the one time in the week we would all sit down to have a meal as a family. During the week my dad worked late so my sister and I would have our tea first around the kitchen table whilst watching the television.

On a Sunday we ate in the dining room, and there was no television, so for me it meant time together as a family, a happy time.

I especially loved my mum's mashed potato, which I would always have more of. This usually meant I was too full to eat dessert; usually rice pudding or semolina; nevertheless, I was made to eat some of the pudding, even though I felt I was full.

Now, as an adult, I still love Sunday dinners and mashed potato, however, when it comes to desserts like rice pudding or semolina, I don't eat these at all, undoubtedly this links back to me being made to eat these puddings as a child.

Making the links

I was obviously not aware of this thought process as it was sub-conscious and automatic until I began my own therapy. That's when I really started thinking about things and making the links, and asking myself, why is it I never fancy these types of puddings when on the whole I love desserts? What I realized was that my experience as a child, of being forced to eat these puddings had put me off them.

Interestingly though my sister had a different experience, she favoured the puddings more than the mashed potato, and now as an adult she still enjoys these types of pudding.

Emotionally Sunday dinners were, for the most part, a happy time for me, so much so that I decided that when I got married we would always make time to have *all* our main meals together, not just on a Sunday because I saw this as an important thing for me. I am aware now that this clearly links to my memories of mealtimes and food when I was a child. I did not like mealtimes without my dad and enjoyed mealtimes better when we all ate together.

Hopefully you can see now how *my* feelings in terms of food, both happy and sad, have had a big influence on my eating habits in the present, my likes and dislikes, and the above is only one example of this.

This example shows how, for me, one of my earliest memories of food was linked with emotions, which in turn influenced my decisions, sub-consciously, as an adult. You need to become aware of these 'links' so you can begin to understand your relationship with food. Once you bring links into your awareness you can then choose to do something different, or at least you will have an understanding of what food 'means' to you, other than just being nutrition.

If you wish, you can take your exercise further and perhaps recall other incidents in your past in terms of food and establish the links.

You can change

It is important at this stage to know that things can be changed and patterns can be changed, we can choose to do something different. Often change can feel uncomfortable at first because it is not familiar to us but if we persevere through this, the change can become the norm and familiar.

Change is often not easy but it is achievable and this is something I really want you to start believing, even if you don't change your diet *you can change the way you feel about yourself* and know **you are ok.**

Often if we make a shift in our thinking the behaviours we do that are self destructive, like over or under-eating will change because we are valuing ourselves more and will therefore look after ourselves more because we now believe we deserve to.

Becoming aware that you have a relationship with food

We are often not aware of how we actually have a relationship with food. A lot of people talk about being 'addicted' to food but tend to overlook the reasons why; they just think that's the way they are. It also does not help that many foods today do contain ingredients in them that are addictive. However I do not believe this is the main reason why people become addicted to food otherwise everyone would be.

I would argue food addiction is mainly emotional and psychological, emerging over a period of time but often having its root causes in childhood; and I believe that by understanding this you can develop strategies to change your relationship with food to a more healthy one.

This is *not* about dieting. If we begin to understand our behaviour with food, and the need it is filling within us, we can fulfill that need in a much healthier way, which will have a positive impact within us and on how we choose to use food within our lives.

I also believe that if we really started to pay attention to our body it *will* tell us what it needs, not just in terms of food and we will begin to get the balance right over other aspects of our lives.

Your Body is Amazing

Our bodies are amazing 'machines' and they will, if allowed, look to attain an *ideal* weight that's right for *us*. This is not about trying to look like the images of people presented to us in magazines because they are not real in the sense that they have been air brushed, touched up etc. Any person seen on the cover of a magazine is extremely likely to look different in the flesh.

I'm not saying there are no beautifully 'slim' people out there, but we are all unique individuals, with bodies unique to us. So isn't it about time we embraced this and began to love *our* bodies and us, rather than getting caught up in the media 'stereotype' circus of everybody being expected to look a certain way. How boring is that?

Can you imagine if 'someone' suggested we should all behave a certain way and there was only one way to *be* that was seen as acceptable in society? There would be an outcry, yet we appear to have no problem with constantly trying to achieve a body image that 'someone' has decided is *the* image.

What is the difference? Just as we are all individuals as people so we are all individuals in appearance. So feel good about your body and your differences you are beautiful inside and out.

Now that we have taken a brief look at what our past relationship with food is, and are starting to understand where some of our current behaviours come from we can begin to take a more in-depth look at how our childhood connection with food is still affecting us now as adults. From there we can consider how you might begin to do something different with food and with your life in general.

Chapter 5

Exploring your addiction

The next two chapters are probably going to be the most challenging and will require some effort on your part, and you must be totally honest with yourself, but if you do manage to stay with it you *will* begin to make sense of your eating habits, and then have some choices to do things differently, if you want to.

Firstly it is important that you begin to view yourself as having an attachment and a relationship to food because then your patterns of eating will begin to make more sense. When we have no attachment or relationship to something we are generally not bothered, and do not invest a lot of our time or effort into whatever it is, we can usually take it or leave it.

However, when we are attached or in a relationship with something or someone then it's a very different story, we are bothered, we invest energy, and generally we are emotionally connected in some way. Which is why talking about food can be a very emotive topic, and can bring up all sorts of different feelings, emotions and memories for people.

If you begin to see yourself as having a relationship with food you can then begin to understand your emotional reaction and the responses you have to it.

In the next chapter I am going to ask you to do an exercise that will take you a week to complete and will involve keeping a diary of what you eat, but firstly we need to explore whether you feel you are ready emotionally to begin to take responsibility for your life and make the commitment to change.

Being responsible can seem frightening

Taking responsibility back for yourself is scary, as you eventually realize that you cannot control anyone else, or how they will react to you. All you can do is control yourself and your choices. However taking responsibility gives you your power back over your life, and the control to do what *you* want to do and to change what *you* want to change, rather than waiting for something or someone else.

You *can* become the person you want to be, but only *you* can make it happen.

I think it is vital when undertaking anything challenging that you have the support of friends and family, while remembering only *you* can change you and do what needs to be done because only *you* know what you really want.

So it is important if you choose to do the exercise to get support, since it may bring up emotions or feelings for you and you *will* need people who can be there for you. This does not mean you *must* share with them, any more than you feel comfortable with, but just that you have people there to turn to if needed.

Now the difficult bit YOU MUST BE TOTALLY HONEST.

The exercise will only work if you are truthful

Many people when talking about weight tend to minimize or maximize what they eat. This may not necessarily be deliberate; it may just be a subconscious way of avoiding something we don't wish to face.

If we want to 'ignore' we have a problem that we *are* able to do something about, we change the information going into our brain so that it 'fits in' with us believing we are powerless in that situation, when actually we are not.

Example

Let's say we're asked, "What have you had to eat today?" When we answer we may subconsciously forget to include snacks we've had, or we 'forget' to remember all the times we finished off what the kids didn't eat etc. People who are underweight may say they have had more food than they actually did by omitting that they actually left most of it. Thus believing they are eating enough when this is in fact not the case.

By doing this we do not get a true picture of what is going on, so when we realize we're putting weight on we fail to make the connection, and again look to lay the blame somewhere else. Saying things like "oh my metabolism must have slowed down" or 'I don't understand how I've managed to put on weight, I've hardly eaten anything". When the reality is we would be able to see the problem, and address it, if only we were totally honest with ourselves.

While it is true that our metabolism slows down as we get older, this should not account for weight gain because we to slow down as we get older meaning we need less food not more. If we are using up less energy we need less calories and our appetite will be reduced. The same as if we start doing lots of physical activity we need more food and will have an increased appetite because our bodies will need more fuel to burn.

By letting ourselves only know the 'half truth' we leave ourselves very little option to do something different, and consequently end up believing there is nothing we can do about it. So we stay the way we are, which is fine if we *are happy* with that, but if we are not it can cause problems, leaving us trapped and feeling powerless.

Hence the current 'blame culture'. People waiting for someone else to take responsibility, when really it is up to the individual to be responsible for themselves. As adults we are not accountable for anyone else or their actions, (our children being the exception) *but we are accountable for our actions and ourselves.*

I understand this may be a hard concept for many to grasp, especially in today's society, but it's one that is essential if you want to do anything to change your life. If you wait for other people you may be waiting forever. Most people who get on in life do so because they take control. They are not waiting for something, or someone else to do it for them, and they don't give up when they have set backs. They recognize these are a part of life and not personal to them. Everyone has problems and ups and downs; it is how they are dealt with that makes the difference.

For example after a bad day at work you can choose to dive into the fridge and comfort eat or you can choose to have a relaxing bath.

Which is why it is really important to be honest or the exercise will not work, and you will limit your options. The thing to remember is that if you are not honest the only person it really affects is you. No one else has to read the diary it is just for you.

The diary is not about giving yourself a hard time over what you are eating, or using it to feel bad about yourself. It is about making sense of your relationship with food and understanding it better, so *you* can make it a healthier relationship, and give yourself options.

You need to choose how you want to do the exercise

You will need a small pad and a pen, and you must carry these around with you wherever you go. How you choose to write things down is up to you. You may want to devise a table or just make notes. It doesn't matter, and whatever works best for you is more likely to ensure you complete the exercise properly.

By doing the exercise for yourself and by you deciding

how you write it down, it shows that you are actually making a commitment meaning you are more likely to complete the exercise, and gain a sense of personal achievement when you do so.

It often feels easier to let people do things for us and there can be a desire to look to others for the answers but we have to decide for ourselves whether or not we want to do the exercise and if we do, how we want to make it work for us.

So I will explain what I want you to do and then you can decide how you prefer to do it. There is no point in me telling you how best to do it because that may only be the best way for me. What works for one person may not necessarily work for someone else. If I devise a chart some people will like it, others may be put off by it, and so by doing it the way that works best for you, you are already making it easier for yourself, and are more likely to stick to it.

This is about *you* taking control and making decisions for yourself about *your* life, I can guide you, but I cannot do it for you, the work needs to come from you.

You may not feel ready

If you find yourself putting off the exercise, and coming up with excuses, take some time to think what this might be about. Ask yourself questions like:

What might I be avoiding?

What is this bringing up for me that I may not want to face or deal with?

What purpose, if any, does it serve in my life for me to stay this way?

Am I genuinely happy/content with the way I am?

People are very good at avoiding situations that might be painful for them, or touch things inside them that they do not want to deal with. So if you are struggling with the exercise this may be what is happening for you. If so, *that's fine*, just be aware of it.

It is always harder to choose than to avoid. To choose places the responsibility back with us, we can no longer pretend it is about something out of our control. Our life and choices then come down to us, which means we have to deal with what goes wrong, as well as what goes right.

Dealing with the things we perceive as going right is great, it's dealing with what didn't go as well that's really hard and then it's easier to blame someone or something else.

Again this is *not* about making us feel bad, it's about looking at what happened, where did things go wrong and what could I have done differently. We cannot change the past, so beating ourselves up about it is not the answer, all that will do is make you feel worse, and then you will probably go and binge eat, and feel even worse, and so on, as a result the cycle of an unhealthy relationship with food starts all over again.

Just pick yourself up and appreciate that you're human, you are not perfect, and no one is.

Try to learn from what went wrong, because the one thing you can do is change *your* future in terms of *your* relationship with food or anything else for that matter. The way it is now does not have to be the way it is forever, you *do* have the control. So when you do this exercise make sure you are not just using it as a means to look at what you eat, so you can make yourself 'not ok', and end up staying where you are (avoiding).

Changing *any* relationship is hard. Just take a minute to think about someone close to you and the relationship you have with him or her, and how that relationship is. I'm sure that you can remember times when the relationship has been hard work; times when you may have felt you had had enough.

I'm also confident that for the most part you get a lot out of the relationship, largely due to the effort you have made, and continue to make, to keep the relationship healthy. We often do not stay in relationships that have become unhealthy because they are not good for us and we can become ill and depressed if we do stay in them.

So why do we continue with an unhealthy relationship with food, that in due course also often makes us ill and depressed? Why do we not change it? The reason is clear; *something else is going on for us rather than just the food we are eating.* Hopefully this exercise will begin to help you find out what that something is.

So if you choose to do the exercise you must be honest.

If you choose not to do the exercise its fine read the rest of the book if you want to, if not put it away, you may come back to it another time when you are more ready. Being willing to challenge ourselves and face up to things we may have been avoiding for years is a very difficult process. I know because having my own therapy has been the hardest thing I've ever done. Equally it's also been the most rewarding.

The most important thing is to know whatever you decide you are still a good person, having an issue with food and our weight does not make you a bad person.

Once you have chosen to continue you are ready to start.

Chapter 6

The Exercise

I want you to keep a food diary for a week; this will not be like other food diaries you may have tried in the past because the emphasis this time is on;

What was going on for you emotionally around the food, and how you felt in terms of what you were eating?

You're going to learn about your relationship with food, when you eat and why, so you can begin to change things. It is *not* about you looking at the diary and thinking, "I'm bad for eating this, and this, and this".

The food *is* important, but more in terms of what it tells you about your relationship with food, rather than how much or what you ate.

When choosing the week to do the exercise it is best to pick a normal week, rather than one when you are on holiday, etc. because you want an average picture of what goes on in your life with food in 'everyday' scenarios. Holidays are to some extent 'irregular' scenarios because people always tend to eat a little differently when on holiday.

What you need to do

What I want you to do is write down EVERYTHING you eat every day of the week, and please be honest with yourself. Even if it's one chip of your child's plate, or someone offers you a single biscuit or sweet, you need to write it down. If you think to yourself "oh that won't matter" chances are it will matter *a lot* so put it down.

Writing down everything you eat is the easy part; the challenging part is to answer the questions in chapter seven in relation to what you write down. This part will take the most time, but it will also be the most useful for you in gaining an awareness of how you use food within your life, and how you might want to change it. If done properly it will hopefully enable you to re-evaluate your relationship and attachment to food.

It doesn't really matter in what order you answer the questions (except question 1) as long as you answer them all. If you are really struggling with a question just make a note and come back to it.

Do try and stay with the question for a little while and think what it is about this particular question that may be challenging for you to answer. What might you have to confront if you answer it?

This may be demanding because if something is out of our awareness we do not at that point have any other options because the knowledge we need is in our subconscious. Once we bring knowledge into our conscious awareness it becomes totally different. We may still choose to do nothing but it will now be a conscious choice we are making.

Example

I may be feeling down so I automatically go for comfort food because at this point I am not aware of the link between my emotion and the food. Once I become aware (which is hopefully what will happen for you through doing the diary), I then have a choice to either go for food or think about what I really need and how to get that need met.

When doing the diary you *must* eat as you normally would otherwise it will not work, if you limit yourself because really you do not want to look at what you are eating, it will not give you a true reflection of your relationship and attachment to food.

The change will come from the diary; so if you find you stop eating certain foods because you have to write them down, again you may be avoiding things that you do not what to face. If you realize this is the case, you may need to stop the exercise and return to it at a later date.

Also if you have a lot going on in your life, this may not be a good time to examine your relationship with food, and the issues this may bring up for you. Only *you* can decide if you're ready and if now is the right time.

However, when deciding if you are ready, you honestly have to ask yourself 'am I just avoiding, or refusing to accept that I have an unhealthy relationship with food?'

As mentioned earlier we can be very good at believing the reason we tell ourselves we 'cannot' try something, even though on some level we will know it's not the *real* reason.

Try using the phrase **I won't** rather than **I can't** because I won't means it's your decision which it is, where as I can't implies there's something external stopping us. THE REALITY IS IT IS US THAT STOPS US FOR WHATEVER REASON.

It is probably best to start the diary on a Monday, rather than a weekend because like holidays sometimes we eat differently on a weekend, or perhaps go out. Also there is something about being back in the 'routine' of the week that may make it easier to remember to keep up the diary.

Then hopefully by the time the weekend comes around you will have become accustomed to carrying a pad and pen everywhere, and writing everything down, making you less likely to forget to take them with you Saturday and Sunday.

Pick a book that fits in your bag or pocket and that's easy for you to take everywhere with you, and then you have no excuses for not filling it in.

Remember to write everything down, and ask the questions for everything, even if it seems futile or pointless. Hopefully it will start to make sense and patterns will begin to emerge as the week progresses. Remember be honest!

As soon as you think you are feeling hungry and are

going to have something to eat you need to answer question no 1, 'How am I feeling at this moment or in general today' which is in capitals. This question needs to be answered before any of the others. It is then not as important what order the other questions are answered in.

The reason for this is the whole point of doing the exercise is to establish if you're eating links into your emotions and you won't be able to do this unless you know how you were feeling either at that moment or in general that day.

For example when you look back over the week you may find the days you felt particularly angry, stressed, sad, tired etc may be the days you ate more and ate more comfort foods, such as chocolate. This would begin to suggest there is a link for you between food and your emotional well-being and you are in some way trying to meet some of your emotional needs through food.

Chapter 7

The Questions

1. HOW AM I FEELING AT THIS MOMENT AND OR IN GENERAL TODAY?

I.e. stressed, tired, flat, empty, nothing, angry, hungry, frightened, sad, happy etc.

2. What time is it?

I.e. lunchtime, breakfast, 10 am, 2.15pm, 9.10pm, etc

3. Where am I?

I.e. desk at work, home in the kitchen, in the car, at a restaurant, etc

4. What am I going to eat?

I.e. chips, mars bar, digestive biscuits, boiled sweet, kid's left-overs, sandwich, lunch etc.

5. How do I feel while I am eating?

I.e. happy, comforted, satisfied, enjoying taste, good, bad etc

6. How do I feel now I have eaten?

I.e. more energy, happy, guilty, full, bad, good, nothing etc

7. Why do I think I have just eaten?

I.e. bored, hungry, it was lunch time, needed a break, tired, stressed etc

The last question may seem a silly one because most people would say I ate because I was hungry but if you are looking to find out if some of your eating has emotional links you need to start getting a sense of the real reason you have eaten.

The reality is in our society, it is unlikely that any of us have ever experienced real hunger, so a lot of the time when we choose to eat it will not actually be because we are really hungry and needing to fill a biological need, the need to live and survive.

For example, if its 2.30pm and you had lunch at 1pm it is unlikely that you will be hungry so if you are feeling the need to eat something what is that about?

Example:

How am I feeling at this moment and or in general?

Fed up and low.

What time is it?

11am

Where am I?

At my desk at work

What am I going to eat?

Mars bar

How do I feel while I'm eating?

Comforted, less fed up

How do I feel now I have eaten?

Guilty, and even more fed up

Why do I think I have just eaten?

Not sure felt low just wanted something nice for me.

Write it down straight away

You should try and write things down as they are happening for you, in terms of what you are eating, otherwise you will not get a true picture of what's happening. Often when we look back at things after an event we may see them in a different way, so it is vital to get down how you are feeling at the time, even if it's only one word. As soon as you know you are going to eat something think about how you are feeling at that moment and write it down.

You may find you are writing 'hungry' all the time, but chances are if you look back and you're eating a lot, there is a good chance your hunger is emotional rather than physical. As a rule we just tend to 'assume' we're hungry, and yet, for probably around 50% of the time we eat for reasons other than hunger. You need to find out what these reasons are.

As you are eating, try not to let thinking about how you feel detract from the effect the food is having on you. If you find this is happening, and you are just not enjoying your food like you used to, give yourself back the permission that it's *ok* to enjoy eating whatever it is you are eating.

This exercise is *not* about you giving yourself a hard time, I'm sure you do enough of that already. It is simply to enable you to become aware of how you use food so you have a choice to change if you want to.

You may find keeping the diary hard

I do realize keeping the food diary may be demanding, especially if you are working, have children etc. So I have kept the questions to a minimum, as shown in the previous example there isn't a great deal of writing involved. The most difficult thing will probably be recognizing how you feel.

If you are really struggling, the most important question to answer, in terms of your feelings is no 1 "how were you feeling *before* you ate" because this may be the key to *why* you are eating, and if it was an emotional need rather than a physical hunger. Your answers will hopefully begin to enable you to see what type of relationship you have with food, and more importantly, how unhealthy it may be.

If possible answer all the questions

It is important to try and answer all the questions if you

can, because as mentioned earlier we are very good at avoiding things we may find difficult to face. Sometimes we can go on making excuses forever, but I believe by choosing this book you must on some level want to change things in your life. So trust your 'instinct' and give it a go, and by doing so you are giving yourself the chance to change.

Sometimes you might not have enough time during the day due to other commitments such as work to spend on the exercise. If so you may want to look over your answers when you have more time, and reflect back on what was happening, and how you were feeling, which is fine. Don't change anything, but if you wish you could add to it, just highlight the bits you are adding *after* the event. This is to make sure you get an accurate picture of your relationship to food.

At the end of each day I also want you to ask yourself how you were feeling 'overall' in relation to *you*, not the food you ate, i.e. depressed, happy, sad, tired, guilty etc. When answering this question note how intense the feeling was.

Doing this will help you see if generally when you are feeling a certain way you crave certain types of food, and if you crave them more the more intense the feeling is. Later on you can begin to make links and start to consider what you may *actually* need when you feel a certain way, instead of food.

You will need to re-learn how to meet your needs

Often as adults we have to learn to meet our own needs in new and different ways from what we are used to. Ways that will be more beneficial to us. This is a difficult process because it often involves re-learning and getting rid of our outdated strategies that may have been useful once upon a time, usually in our childhood when we needed to adapt to a particular environment, but now we need to replace those strategies with new ones that are more useful to us as adults.

It may be helpful at this point to go back and remind yourself of what you realized in chapters three and four. Remember how your relationship with food developed as a child, what your unmet needs were, and what food meant in your family, so you can refresh your memory of the strategies you developed as a child in order to fit in, and how some of these link to food.

Example

Recently I had been watching a film and it stirred up memories and feelings for me, in relation to my mum's death, and I began to get upset. Due to having had my own personal therapy, I was aware of feeling sad and I was able to make the link that this was about my mum dying, but that still didn't stop me from feeling empty inside, and wanting *something* to make me feel better.

So I made myself a cheese and ham toasty, but once it was made I found I didn't really fancy it, and it didn't taste how I wanted it to, so I ended up throwing half of it away. I then had a big bowl of cereal, but did not enjoy this either. Finally my husband went to the shop and brought me some chocolate, because, I just felt I needed something nice, something comforting. The chocolate didn't do the job either and in fact it actually didn't even taste nice. Afterwards, I not only still felt sad and empty, but on top of that I also felt angry with myself because I had eaten so much when in reality I wasn't even hungry and most importantly nothing could bring my mum back.

The reality was it wouldn't have mattered what I had eaten, or done for that matter, because nothing was going to change the fact my mum had died. I needed to grieve for her which means allowing myself to have my feelings, however painful, not trying to avoid them.

Even when I was choosing to eat I knew what I was doing, I knew that I was trying to fill an emotional need, and even said so to my husband, but I still did it. My sadness did not go away because what I really wanted was my mum, and nothing I did, or ate, was going to bring her back.

I needed to let myself have my 'natural' feelings over what had happened and just be sad, granted it's not a nice feeling, but it won't kill me. If you look at it rationally, feelings are an essential part of life and us. They are what enable us to be different and unique, yet we still try so hard to avoid the ones that are painful. My sadness just showed how much I love and miss my mum, which is a very natural process since we were very close.

We need to understand that feelings won't kill us, they may be painful but they can't hurt us physically, and to have them is essential in order for us to be healthy, emotionally as well as physically.

My example shows how easily we can be pulled towards food when we are feeling certain ways, and even though I have a lot of awareness about myself, and knew my need wasn't food, I still ate, so that shows us just how hard it is to stop using food in a negative way, but it is not impossible.

For me, the example I have given is quite extreme in terms of using food in an emotional way; for the most part we use it in much smaller ways, usually out of awareness. If we can bring how we use food in this way into our awareness by doing the exercises, we then have a choice to do something different and we can begin to make little changes, which eventually, will lead to big changes.

Remember if we skim a small pebble across the water it will create a ripple effect, try to skim a boulder across the water and it will just make a big splash and immediately sink to the bottom.

Meaning if we try to make too big a change, it becomes un-maintainable and we 'sink'. However, if we make small manageable changes, they will have a ripple effect in our lives, like the pebble and permanent change becomes much more likely.

Chapter 8

Understanding your addiction to food.

We can now start to look at what the exercise you did in the previous chapter has told you about your relationship with food. On some level you have probably already realized you have an unhealthy relationship with food, otherwise you would not have bought this book. What may surprise you more is just how *much* your relationship with food is linked to how you feel, and to what you eat.

Almost certainly it will be fairly new for you to think about food in terms of a relationship, rather than *just* food, though hopefully after doing the exercises you are perhaps much more aware of this concept, and how it fits into your life.

You will be pleased to know the changes I am discussing do not involve any diets, or even the word diet, or any weighing of yourself, in fact it is probably better that you avoid scales all together, usually all they do is make you feel worse.

We all know one of the main reasons diets don't work is that they are just not maintainable; the only way to change *anything* permanently is to make it livable within *our* lifestyles, not the lifestyle of someone else. This means only *you* know if something is workable in *your* life and if you can live with it permanently. It does not matter if it's livable in any one else's life *only in yours* because everyone is different so what works for you may not be what works for anyone else.

So we're back to it being *your* responsibility to choose things *you* can live with in *your* life. Do not set yourself up to fail by making something unachievable.

Example

I love chocolate and I don't *want* to live without it, if I told myself "I can never have chocolate again" I would be setting myself up to fail, because for me to never again have something I really enjoy eating, would be unachievable. I would only end up feeling bad because I'd had chocolate when I shouldn't have, and probably just end up eating more.

That's not to say I have chocolate every day, because the truth is, since I stopped making it a 'forbidden' food, and allowed myself to know it's ok to have it whenever I want it, I don't actually want it half as often.

Once again this refers back to having a relationship with food, because in relationships we have all sorts of feelings happiness, sadness, guilt, fear, anger, etc. so this is true if we have a relationship with food, especially one that's unhealthy.

When we make something forbidden we also make it bad

When I make a food forbidden, and bad, I associate a certain feeling with it, meaning when I eat that food I end up associating the feeling to me, so I end up feeling bad. I am confident that at some stage most of you will have ended up feeling awful/guilty etc after eating things like chocolate, crisps or a cheeseburger.

The truth is, no 'food' alone is bad for you we only make it bad for us when we eat too much of it and this can also be true for 'healthy' foods. If all someone ate was lettuce, even though as a general food group it is considered healthy, it too would become unhealthy because lettuce alone would not give us enough of what we need to have a healthy balance. A cheeseburger once a month is not unhealthy if we combine it with a healthy balance of other food throughout the month.

So our relationship with our diet becomes double edged, not only do we associate certain foods as good and bad, but we then also choose the so-called 'bad' foods when we are trying to use food to fill an emotional need. The result is we end up feeling twice as bad, bad because we have chosen what we perceive as a 'wrong food' and bad because that food didn't fill the emotional need anyway, and it never will. At best all food can do is fill us when we are physically hungry.

Plus most foods we choose to fill our emotional needs tend to be the ones with the least nutrients, the ones least likely to fill our hunger meaning we often end up eating more.

We need to stop labelling foods as good or bad

We must stop labelling food as 'good' or 'bad'. FOOD IS JUST FOOD. It's what *we* choose to do with it that determines whether our relationship with it is healthy or unhealthy.

There is something very liberating about not labelling food, but it is not an easy thing to do. Society has almost 'brainwashed' us into thinking certain foods are bad and other foods are good, often making us feel that if we eat those 'bad' foods we must be bad, and the people who eat the 'good' foods must be good, or better, than those of us who eat more of the 'bad' foods.

Unfortunately I cannot change society, but what I can do is enable you to see that regardless of what you eat *you* are *ok*. Food does not define the person you are on the inside, even if it may restrict you outwardly.

I remember being 'overweight' and wanting to be thinner (I use the commas because I was only 'overweight' in terms of how society expected me to look; it was *never* a health issue). I decided, as so many of us have, to diet. However, I didn't follow a diet as such; I just decided to cut out certain 'unhealthy' foods.

Sadly, what happened then was I started to obsess about the foods I felt I could not have. I would long for chocolate or cakes, and spend ages looking at them, torturing myself, because I knew they were forbidden. When I did succumb to one of my 'forbidden' foods I would feel awful, and guilty, I felt like I had let myself down.

This went on for a long time, with me thinking that if I could just shift half a stone I would be happy, and giving myself a really hard time because I couldn't do it. The reality was that losing the weight had absolutely nothing to do with whether I was happy or not, but it took me having my own therapy to realize this.

Being content with ourselves comes from within us not from what we look like

My happiness, or as I prefer to call it, contentment, because we cannot be happy all of the time comes from within me. We can be content within ourselves, whilst being sad, or whilst things in life are not quite going how we had hoped. This level of contentment comes with knowing that whatever happens, *we are ok*.

Once I realized my contentment came from within *me,* and not from some external force, like money, or how I looked, my relationship with food changed. I was no longer trying to find contentment in my appearance, and my weight has now remained the same for several years, give or take a pound or two.

I eat what I want, when I want. The difference for me now is that I don't think of foods as wrong or right, and I no longer associate how I'm feeling with what I am eating. I eat because I am hungry or because I fancy something. I don't forbid myself anything; I just listen to what my body really needs and by doing so I maintain a healthy weight.

I am not, nor will I ever be stick thin, I am curvy and that's great, it's how I am meant to be, and the more comfortable I feel with me as a person, the more comfortable I feel within my body.

Having a healthy relationship with food means I don't fancy cakes or chocolate every day, because for the most part I get my emotional needs met in different ways, and do not associate the food I eat with how I feel, I manage to keep them separate.

That is not to say I don't enjoy my food, I love food, but it's not the same kind of love I have in relationships with people, it is not a love that can hurt me or cause me pain, that can only happen if *we* give food that power.

We can control our relationship with food

Unlike being in a relationship with a person, where we cannot control them, or how they respond to us, we *can* control food; it is not a real living entity with feelings. *We* give food the feelings, so ultimately *we* make ourselves feel good or bad, in terms of what we eat.

I gave an example in the last chapter of a time recently when I used food in an unhealthy way, and I think that's important because even though the majority of the time I now have a healthy relationship with food, there are times when I still turn to food to give me comfort, even when I am aware that is what I am doing.

We're human beings, we cannot be prefect, and at times of stress we will be drawn back into our old ways of coping. This is natural, and it's not about giving ourselves a hard time when we do. The more awareness we have the better, because at least we then have the choice to do something different and get our needs met in a more beneficial way.

In my example I knew what I was doing and *choose* to do it anyway. What I didn't then do was give myself a hard time over it, nor did I make the food good or bad. I just ate what I felt I needed. Ultimately the food did not make me feel any better, and I knew it wouldn't and couldn't, but it did not make me feel worse either because *I did not give the food that power.* I did what I did and it was ok and I am still ok.

Chapter 9

We get caught in a negative cycle with food

Initially the food does work as a distraction, and it tastes good, but soon after eating it we are troubled by guilt and end up feeling worse than we did initially. The cycle then starts all over again, feeling down, fed up, lonely etc – eat - feeling worse – eat more.

This cycle becomes harder and harder to break and in the mean time we never actually get our real need met. Eventually we begin to think less and less of ourselves for not being able to do anything about it and so we eat more to comfort ourselves and so it goes on.

Our relationship with food becomes a damaging one; we abuse ourselves with food and end up having little respect for our health or ourselves. Before you know it your whole life is revolving around food, and you don't have time to have your feelings over anything else except food. Once food becomes an 'addiction' it will take over your life so you don't have to face anything because there will be no room in your life for anything but your addiction.

That is what addictions do; they engulf you and leave no room for anything else. They become your main relationship superceding everything else in your life.

This is very sad because ultimately we are all ok, but somewhere along the way we have forgotten this, and we need to get this belief back.

When we start to begin to feel positive within ourselves the food *will* become less and less of an issue because we will begin to have a healthy relationship with ourselves. Our unhealthy relationship with food ultimately mirrors our unhealthy relationship with ourselves because when we believe we are not ok we do not look after ourselves properly emotionally or physically.

Once we believe we are ok it becomes natural to look after ourselves. We would never deliberately hurt someone we cared for, yet when we have an unhealthy relationship with food we are in due course hurting ourselves, emotionally and physically.

We need to learn to nurture ourselves

We need to re-learn how to take care of ourselves and cherish who we are. That is why this book is not about dieting or looking a certain way it is about caring for *us*, and once we can do this properly our bodies will find their natural weight. This will be different for everyone because we are all unique and it's time we started being proud of this rather then trying to fit into some stereotypical image.

How to make changes

When looking back over the exercise you did in Chapter 7 it is important not to make yourself good or bad, or associate the food as good or bad, it is about making links between what you eat and how you feel, so you can then look to do something different, if you want to.

Just remember food is not the enemy and you are fine regardless.

So get out the diary you kept for the week and go through it, asking yourself the following question.

"What was the 'feeling / need' I think I was trying to fill with food?"

It's unlikely you will have been filling an emotional need every time you ate, obviously there will be times when you ate merely because you were hungry, however, there may also have been times when you were hungry and trying to fill an emotional need as well.

You will probably be able to tell by the food you picked, often when eating is about meeting an emotional need, rather than actually being hungry, we tend to pick foods we believe give us comfort, for example chocolate, cakes, crisps, take-aways, etc, and it doesn't help that a lot of these foods are deliberately made to be more 'addictive' than healthier options. What then happens is eating this kind of food becomes a habit or part of our routine and we lose track of the reason we were eating it in the first place.

It's really important to go through *all* the foods you ate each day to try and get a sense of how you use food in your life and to begin to understand the relationship you have with food. Initially it may be difficult to know what *'feeling'* or *'need'* you were trying to fill, hopefully this is where the diary will help, as you should already have written down how you were feeling before you ate.

So the example I gave for the diary was I thought I was just feeling fed up so I ate a chocolate bar, but thinking about how I was feeling enabled me to realize I was sad. I had listened to a song on the radio on my way to work, which reminded me of my mum, and because I had avoided the feeling it stayed with me and I tried to feel better by eating. I was trying to avoid my feelings of sadness, rather than allowing myself to experience them. I did not want to stay with them so I tried to distract myself with food rather than look for what I may in fact need at that time.

What might you have needed instead of food?

What else may I have needed at the time instead of, or as well as, food?

Now that you have identified the feeling you may have been trying to fill with the food you can begin to think about what you may *actually* have needed at the time.

If we go back to the example of the mars bar, I identified I was trying to fill my feeling of sadness with food rather than experiencing it. What might I have needed at the time instead of the mars bar to allow me to feel?

Well, because I was sad it would have been helpful

for me to acknowledge those feelings because once I acknowledge them I can then think about what I might be sad about, which then gives me choices to do something about how I am feeling, rather than trying to avoid my feelings through food.

Maybe I just needed to let myself acknowledge I was sad, and in doing so realize food would not make me feel better. Perhaps I may have needed to speak to someone to get some comfort, and just let him or her know I was feeling sad. If I had recognized and acknowledged my sadness I could have taken better care of myself by re-planning my day and managing my work load so as not to make myself feel worse e.g. by not pushing myself, letting myself have a full dinner break, taking breaks when needed, finishing on time, etc.

Sometimes we may not realize how something has affected us because as you now already know we are very good at avoiding painful feelings, hence why we eat for comfort, so in the car when the song came on I may not even have registered I was sad because I was driving and needed to get to work, but my subconscious will. As a result the feeling would probably have stayed with me all day regardless of what I did, or what I ate. My 'need' was to feel sad about my mum and to know that was the appropriate thing to do.

Therefore, thinking about how we are feeling before we eat allows us to really become aware of what is happening for us in our lives emotionally, and what makes us happy, sad, etc. which means we are less likely to miss our feelings, and not keep eating to try and get comfort.

You can train yourself to be aware of how you are feeling

If I had not thought about how I was feeling before I ate the mars bar I would not have realized I was sad, or what I was sad about. So just thinking about my feelings before I eat can give me all that awareness. Obviously training ourselves to think this way does not happen overnight but the more we do it the easier it will become, until it is happening without us having to try.

Eventually you will become aware of the feeling as it happens, so in my example I would have realized what was happening in the car and then been able to decide what I needed other than comfort eating.

It is important to be aware that we will not always feel better quickly when having our feelings, because often we need to stay with those feelings and allow ourselves to acknowledge and express them fully before feeling better. We may also need support from family, friends, or other things, to enable us to do this.

People think food is a quick fix because it gives us an instant gratification, but what we now know is we usually feel worse after, so in the long run using food to meet emotional needs only creates more emotional needs. This in turn results in us eating more to keep avoiding them.

If we can just recognize when our need to eat is not about being hungry by identifying when it is an emotional issue we can then know that eating will not change this, or make it better. Just having this awareness is a big step forward in terms of making your relationship with food a healthier one.

You can, of course, still choose to eat, but you do so in awareness, meaning you can no longer try and blame other things, *it is your responsibility*, and ultimately you make the choices and have to live with the consequences of those choices.

As I said earlier *choosing* to eat for comfort does not make you bad unless you allow it to, but if you are unhappy with the way you are only you can do something about that.

Change takes time so be patient with yourself

It may take you a while to begin to know what you might have needed instead of food, which is normal. It does take time to begin to allow ourselves to really listen to what our bodies need, both emotionally and physically, especially if we have had an unhealthy relationship with food for a long time.

Often it is also hard to face the reality that we need to change and do something different even when we know what we are doing is actually harming us, hence the saying 'ignorance is bliss'. When something is familiar it often feels safe even though we know it is destructive to us, so it can be very hard to change. To change, although beneficial, is to venture into the unknown and the unfamiliar and can feel scary so we stick to what feels familiar despite the often negative consequences.

Take comfort from the fact that you are now more aware of your eating patterns and relationship to food, which, if nothing else, means *you* can choose not to eat for an emotional need, and that alone is a big achievement. Remember little changes can have a big impact on our lives.

Tiredness and hunger

Something to be aware of is if you regularly feel tired, and eat to try and get some energy, because being tired can also be about something else. If you find you are frequently tired and that seems to be the feeling you have when you eat, you really need to be asking yourself; should I be tired?

For example; if you are getting eight hours sleep a night, and sleeping quite well, it is unlikely that you are in fact physically tired, it is more likely that you are holding in the emotions you are again trying to avoid. Holding emotion in is extremely tiring, which is why people who are depressed often feel tired all the time, and sleep a lot.

If you do look at your lifestyle and sleeping pattern, and find how you are living your life is actually why you are always tired, although this is not emotional the awareness enables you to choose to do something different. You can choose to live your life a different way, or, make adjustments so you are not always tired, which ultimately should have an impact on your eating.

Chapter 10

How to meet your need differently

Ask yourself, "How might I meet my need in a different way, or do something different?"

I briefly mentioned some of this in the previous question about what might you have needed instead of food? They do overlap a bit, in that if you identify what you might have needed instead of food this may also give you the answer to what you need to do to begin meeting that need in a different way.

I gave some suggestions of how I might have gotten my sadness met differently rather than through food, while acknowledging the need to have my sadness and that the process was not just about me getting to feel better.

So how might you meet your emotional needs differently? What do you need when you are feeling sad, angry, frightened, happy etc? Often it is hard to recognize how we are feeling and what we might need. Many people are used to avoiding at least some of their emotions so it takes time to start listening to our bodies and realizing what our emotional needs are.

Hopefully by keeping the diary you will at least have begun to have a sense of your emotions, and which of those emotions tends to lead you to eat or use food as a way of avoiding them. Now you have developed this sense, you need to train yourself to listen to what your body might actually need, when it doesn't actually need food.

How do we separate our genuine hunger from our emotional hunger?

As discussed earlier there will of course be times when you are genuinely hungry, but how do you begin to separate your hunger for food from your emotional hunger? Often the two become so confused it is hard to know, especially if our food choices in general have now become unhealthy.

It would be easy if we only ate unhealthy when we were feeling a certain way but often what happens is because a lot of unhealthy food is more addictive we start using it to fill an emotional need and before we know it, it is all, or the majority of what we are eating and so it becomes the norm and we blame the food instead of looking at our choices and taking control.

Food can only control us if we let it, we need to take the control back and make informed choices about what we eat and how we want to be with food.

We all know there are healthy foods and unhealthy foods and we all know which ones are which, but as discussed earlier if we eat in balance then our relationship with food can be healthy and we will still be able to have the things we like in moderation.

Once we fill our emotional needs in a different way, or at least become aware we are using food in this way, we can begin to change and have choices. This is not about saying you can't have this or you must eat that, it is about *you* deciding how you want to be.

When we deny ourselves something we crave it more

Most people are aware that as soon as you tell yourself you can't have something the more you crave it, so what's the point, all you end up doing is torturing yourself and you usually end up eating what you believe to be 'forbidden' anyway.

I used to be like that, I would spend hours looking at sweets and cakes believing I couldn't have them, and as soon as breakfast was over I would be wondering what was for dinner because I believed I shouldn't eat in-between meals, and that I had to be a certain size to be 'ok'.

Once I allowed myself to know it was fine to eat sweets or cakes if I wanted to I found I did not crave them as much and so only tended to eat them in moderation. When I gave up believing I had to be a certain weight to be accepted 'miraculously', I have stayed the same weight and never dieted since. I don't own a pair of scales, what's the point, you know yourself if you are using food in a negative or destructive way.

Being slim does not mean we are healthy

Being a size 8 or 10 does not necessarily mean you are healthy, or that your relationship with food is good. A lot of slim people have big issues with food, but because visually, in terms of society, the way they look fits, they think that's fine, it is only when a slim person becomes visually unpleasing to society i.e. too thin that it becomes an issue, and even then not in the same way it does if society sees you as overweight.

If we eat properly and have a good relationship with food, and ourselves, I believe our bodies will find a 'natural' weight; the problem for people with this is that it often isn't how they want to look because it isn't the figures we are bombarded with in all the magazines we pick up.

Images we see in magazines are not real

Let's just think about this for a minute, the images you see in a magazine photo shoot are not natural. The models and celebrities will have a team of make up artists at their disposal, and if that's not quite good enough the photographer will position them in a way that appears best and adjust the lighting to suit, which makes the model look slimmer. If this still doesn't do the job somebody on a computer will airbrush out any unsightly 'bits' and hey presto they look fabulous. But trust me, so would we if we went through the same process

So why is it we then try and achieve this look, or even believe we can, *it isn't real*. That's not to say there are no models or stars that look good naturally, of course there are, but it's their job. They have to look good all the time that's how they make their living, which is why they have make up artists, personal trainers, often their own chefs and designers; they do not lead 9-5 jobs like the majority of us.

So how can we compare ourselves to them and why would we want to, *we are fantastic as we are*, and often celebrities are not that happy, even with the 'lifestyle' they have they still have their own emotional 'baggage'. Consequently a lot of them end up in rehab for drink or drug problems, and some of them will have their own unhealthy relationships with food, usually in terms of being underweight or having a very inconsistent weight, fluctuating between being underweight to overweight.

We need to learn to accept ourselves

Like it or not we are all born a certain way and we have to learn to accept ourselves for who we are. I am five feet tall and no matter what I do I will never be taller, so I accept this is the way I am and I am fine with it. Constantly wishing I were taller won't help, it will only make me miserable and in fact I love being small and I love myself inside and out as we all can.

This does not mean I am perfect but that I accept all of myself the nice and the not so nice because I know I am a good person and how I look will not change this.

I like many others used to believe if I could just lose

half a stone I would be happy. What a load of rubbish, losing half a stone won't make *me* happy, happiness comes from inside, all losing half stone would have done is make me slimmer. It would not have changed anything else in my life only how I look visually.

If I am not happy on the inside whatever I do on the outside is only a diversion and a way to avoid facing the real reason I am unhappy. That's why a lot of the stars who appear to have everything end up drinking or taking drugs in excess because although they have the money, the fame and the figure this is all superficial and underneath all this, inside, they are frequently fraught with deep-seated problems and insecurities.

Food is easy to misuse

It's easy to misuse food because it is so readily available, we have to eat to live, whereas we don't need to drink alcohol or take drugs to live (medications are another matter). Drugs are also illegal and a lot harder to get hold of. Plus food does not change us to the extent drink and drugs can. We can use food destructively and still go to work, drive and lead a relatively normal life, unless of course our relationship with food has become so unhealthy we are physically restricted in some way.

Unfortunately this means it is also very difficult to change how we manage our diet because we cannot avoid eating in the same way we can avoid drink and drugs. To live we've got to eat. What we may be able to do though is change things in our lives in relation to food.

For example if we have a take-away every week and initially we find it too hard to not have a take-away, we may be able to change what we order to something more healthy, thereby getting the best of both worlds, or limit our takeaways to fortnightly etc until we achieve our healthy balance with food.

We have to look at the bigger picture in terms of what we might need in our life to get our needs met in a healthier way, rather than through food. What might be missing in our lives, and what may need to happen for us to begin to feel more *content*?

I use the word content instead of happy because as mentioned earlier it is unrealistic to think we can be happy all of the time, life is not like that. I think this is where many people go wrong, they aim for happiness all the time and it is an unattainable goal, so when they fall short of this goal, they feel rubbish and then try to meet their need in a different way, or mask the feelings through food, drugs, drink, shopping etc.

When we are content we know even though we may be sad or angry or when things are difficult in our life we will get through and be ok. It is an underlying belief that although life is not always 'hunky dory' we can cope even though we may feel awful. It is usually when trying to avoid these uncomfortable feelings that we look for something else to fill the gap in our lives. Food is such an easy option, rather than staying with what feels uncomfortable and working through it.

The reality is life has 'ups and downs' and we cannot avoid this no matter how hard we try. For example, we are born to lose people we love through death, so life cannot be great all of the time. We need to accept this and learn ways of coping other than diving into the biscuit barrel.

Chapter 11

You need to start looking at the bigger picture

The diary will have helped you become aware of the feelings that you may have been avoiding or trying to meet through food, so this should give you an idea of a theme or pattern in terms of when you eat, which will help you begin to look at the bigger picture in terms of your life.

If you can begin to explore the bigger picture, and your life in general, it is more likely that your choices around food will change permanently. If we only deal with things on a superficial level we often end up reverting back to our old unhelpful ways. Fad diets are one example, because the false belief is if we are thinner we will be happier, but more often than not the weight is used as a diversion from the real problem. We concentrate on this to avoid the real issue.

The real issue is never dealt with so even when we do become slimmer it isn't enough, so we find we are still not content and end up continuing to use food as an emotional crutch. This is why most dieters either put the weight back on or keep it off in an inappropriate way, perhaps by starving themselves or making themselves sick.

We need to look within ourselves to find the answers

You need to look within yourself to begin to understand what is really going on in your life and to find out the reasons you use food in the way you do. *You* will have the answers because no one knows you better than you. It's just that we forget to ask ourselves and instead look to others for the answers. In reality how can someone else have the answers to questions about your life and what you want? As a starting point try asking yourself the following questions

What do you need in your life?

What are you avoiding through food?

What needs to change in your life in terms of how you meet your needs?

What are you not getting?

An example from my own life

I often find I eat when I am feeling stressed and overwhelmed because eating comfort foods like chocolate and crisps does help me feel better initially as it takes my mind of what's going on in my life and enables me to avoid thinking about my stress. But afterwards what have I achieved, I am still stressed and now I also feel guilty for eating. Plus I have done nothing productive to help my situation like getting support or looking at what I might need to change in my life so I am less stressed.

Luckily I am now aware of this so I can usually spot when it's happening to me and as a result I can then choose what I actually need. Sometimes I choose to talk to someone and get support with how I am feeling and even though it can be hard to open up to people and admit I am struggling, it is usually very beneficial, providing I pick a person I know will understand and be empathic. Otherwise I could just end up feeling worse. When I have chosen this option I have always found I feel better and often the person I have confided in also has some good ideas about things I could change or do to be less stressed.

Other times I choose to use relaxation techniques I have learnt such as deep breathing, to calm myself so I am able to think rationally about what is causing my stress and what I can do to improve this. There are also times I choose to eat but the difference is I do this in awareness so it does not become excessive, whilst also knowing there will be changes I need to make in my life so as to reduce my stress. This is really important because stress is one of our biggest killers and can cause illnesses' such as cancer and heart attacks.

What I do not do is try and avoid or replace my stress with food, but equally I know it is fine to treat myself and have nice things. We all need this permission and if used sensibly it can be another way of meeting our own needs and reducing stress.

If you eat for the right reasons you can enjoy food without feeling guilty

I always have something nice in the house that is just for me, it's usually chocolates. I make a coffee and have two or three chocolates with my coffee and it feels great because I love chocolate and when I eat it this way, rather than to try to avoid or fill an emotional need I really enjoy it. There is no guilt because I am no longer in a game with food.

I used to buy chocolate and eat too much really fast, and my friend once said to me "how can you enjoy eating it that way surely you will just end up feeling sick?" Of course she was right. Often if we are eating for the wrong reasons we don't enjoy the food or we get past the enjoyment stage and end up feeling sick or bloated, not to mention the feelings we then have which I touched upon earlier, e.g. guilt.

Have you ever eaten so much of something you think you will never eat it again, a bit like when you have too much to drink, but you soon forget the feeling and end up doing the same thing again and again. Eating food for emotional reasons ultimately is not enjoyable, physically or emotionally, because we often don't know when to stop, we don't want to stop, or we think we can't stop, simply because we are trying to fill a need, or avoid feeling something. *Food cannot fill our emotional needs*. All food can do in terms of filling a need is satisfy our physical hunger. It can never satisfy our emotional hunger.

I am not saying we shouldn't enjoy food, let's face it a lot of food tastes nice and that's great, but we still cannot substitute food, as a way of meeting our emotional needs whatever they are.

We need to be aware that eating is very social

There is also something about *where* and *when* we eat that I think we forget. Eating is very social and often it will be the company we are in and the good time we are having that makes the overall food 'experience' better. The trouble starts when we try and recreate this feeling on our own, through food because we believe it was the food that made us feel good.

If you go back to when you looked at what food meant for you as a child and in terms of your family you may have found a lot of your happy times as a child involved food, for example birthday parties, Christmas etc. You can then begin to see how as a child it is easy to confuse the food with the feelings of happiness you had at these times and so try and recreate that happiness again as an adult through food. Once you understand this and realize it was not the food that created the happy feelings you can begin to find out what you really need to feel happy.

Humans need social contact

We live in an age where it is becoming harder and harder to get the social contact we need as humans, and we are becoming more and more withdrawn into ourselves. No one seems to talk to each other properly any more, partly because we are all so busy, and partly due to certain inventions such as the computer, the mobile phone and I-pods.

Again I am not saying these things are bad but e-mailing and texting is helping to further reduce our contact through social interaction, and we all need this for our emotional well-being. So it becomes more and more difficult to fulfil this need.

Food on the other hand has become so much more accessible, it often seems the easiest option, and it may be in the short term, but we now know having a long term 'unhealthy' relationship with food is not an easy option, and it is a very hard thing to change especially if it becomes an addiction.

Studies done in Romanian orphanages (1) demonstrate how important social contact is for emotional health and how unimportant food can be. What these studies showed were that even when the children had all their basic needs catered for in terms of food, water, shelter and clothing but got no physical contact or significant social interaction they failed to thrive. Thus proving food alone was not enough to sustain them emotionally or physically.

Another example is an experiment carried out with monkeys (2), they placed one 'wire' monkey holding food and one 'cloth' monkey with no food into an environment with real monkeys to see what would happen. What they found was the real monkeys preferred the comfort offered by the 'cloth' monkey rather than the food. I find this very powerful in terms of what we need as humans to be physically and emotionally healthy, contact and stable relationships. Often we ignore our most important needs and then wonder why we are not content in life, and end up turning to food, drugs or drink.

Humans need stable relationships and healthy attachments

If we don't have stable relationships and proper contact we will make relationships with other things, such as food, because this is better than the alternative of facing our void or loneliness, or whatever you want to call it, and if it becomes a full-blown addiction then our main relationship is now with the substance we are addicted to, in this case food, leaving little room for anything else.

To give you an example of how powerful these unhealthy relationships become you just have to look at the number of people who have lost relationships, through addictions, including losing their children, because they are no longer able to care for them or have a healthy relationship with them. Their unhealthy relationship with the 'substance' has taken over.

Letting go of relationships like this means facing painful things that we don't want to face, which is why we avoided them in the first place, and looking into ourselves to find answers and meaning. Addiction creates meaning in our lives but in a destructive way.

We need to begin to create new meaning that is healthy and meets the needs we have, instead of trying to meet our needs through food and, ultimately, failing.

In order to do this we have to really look at our lives closely which may be painful, but unless we can find out what it is that's missing, and fill these needs in more beneficial ways, we will continue our unhelpful patterns with food.

Let's face it having a damaging relationship with food ultimately leads to all sorts of physical and emotional illnesses and it can even be a slow *suicide*. More people die from obesity related illnesses than anything else, even cancer, simply put, many people die from the bad choices they make around food.

This leads us to the next question we need to ask ourselves in order to change our relationship with food, and ultimately change our life.

1) The Science of Mother's Day (1999) *Not Really a Monkey.* (Web Version)
http:/whyfiles.org1087mother/4.html
2) Harlow, H. F. (1958) 'The Nature of Love' *American Psychologist Journal* 13 573-687

Chapter 12

What is missing in my life?

We have already established that if we do tend to use food negatively, we often do so to try to fill an emotional need and to get comfort from rather than because we are physically hungry. Many of us already know we use food in this way but seem to be unable to do anything about it, despite all the diets and information available to us regarding what we should and shouldn't be eating.

I believe this is because unless we know what it is that is missing in our lives or what needs we are trying to fill with food, how can we choose to do something different.

Hopefully the earlier exercises will have given you some idea of what is happening for you emotionally when you eat for comfort and what needs you are trying to fill. With this is mind we now need to look a bit deeper and ask ourselves some difficult questions.

1) What is it that I think is missing in my life?

2) What am I not happy with in my life?

3) What would I like to change in my life?

Spend some time thinking about these questions and then write down your answers as this will give you a starting point of how to begin getting what you need and making your life how you want it to be, so that you no longer need to use food in an emotional / unhealthy way.

Food can never fill an emotional need, the only need food can fill is a physical hunger.

I believe if you are happy with *you* and content within yourself you would not then eat for comfort to the extent of it becoming an addiction and unhealthy. We all get down at times because life is filled with disappointments and upsets, as well as good times, but if someone is genuinely content within themselves they are more able to manage these ups and downs whilst staying balanced. In other words it would not lead to an addiction with food, or anything else for that matter.

Everyone at some point comfort eats but the difference is if you feel good within yourself you keep the balance, and food does not become your crutch because you are not trying to fill an internal need with an external substance. Once the balance tips and the food becomes tied in with your emotions you are in a no win situation.

When this happens we feel we have to keep eating because only when we are eating do we feel better, but it's a false feeling of happiness that goes soon after we stop eating, resulting in you feeling the need to eat some more. Then what you learn is to eat every time you are down, sad, frustrated, scared, angry, etc. rather than having those feelings, and looking into what they are really about and what you might need at that time to help you. Hence people talk about never feeling full. You will never feel full if you are trying to use food to fill an emotional void, its an impossibility, you are not hungry for food you are hungry for something else, the key is to find out what.

What is missing is the fundamental belief that we are worthwhile

I believe people generally get an unhealthy relationship with food because on some level they do not feel worthwhile and 'good enough'. If you genuinely believed you were ok you would not treat your body with the lack of respect and nurturing that often comes from a bad relationship with food.

I find it really sad when people are putting their health and well being at risk and in some cases are even committing slow suicide through food. Ask yourself this question 'would you really do that to yourself if you were truly content and felt good about yourself'? It's almost as if you're punishing yourself through food, as if you don't deserve any better. If someone wants to take their own life we often think that person must be feeling really depressed or must have some serious problems going on in their lives, yet if someone is eating themselves to death, albeit slowly, people see this differently. Why is it any different with food?

You cannot think much about yourself if you treat your body in such a way, anyone who loved him or herself would not mistreat their body in this way. You would not wish illness on anyone you loved yet by having an unhealthy relationship with food we can bring illness upon ourselves, and often suffering to those around us who then have to care for us or deal with our unhappiness.

The harsh reality is that feeling worthwhile only comes from within, from you learning to love yourself. It cannot come from food or any other external thing. There is no doubt we would feel better initially if we lost weight but our emotional issues would remain, unless we deal with them. This is why when some people win a lot of money they find it does not make them as happy as they thought it would. The only thing money can do is sort money problems; it cannot deal with emotional issues or low self worth. Likewise losing weight can make you look a different way but if there are other emotional issues going on being slimmer cannot sort those and neither can money, drugs, drink etc.

If they could then no one in the world who was slim or rich would ever be unhappy and as we know that definitely is not the case, if anything it often makes people worse because they realize it hasn't made them happy. What you need to do is to start looking into yourself and how you start loving and nurturing you, so you feel worthwhile and valued.

Exercise

Learning to love and nurture yourself can be hard, it took me a long time and a lot of my own therapy to get there, but here is an exercise that will help.

Part one

Everyday I want you to find something positive about yourself or what you have done and write it down. You can write more than one if you feel able to and over time I want you to build up to five things each day. When this becomes easy and you really believe what you are writing you are well on your way to feeling good about yourself.

Examples

'I like the way my hair looks today.'

'I managed that difficult situation at work really well today.'

'I cooked a lovely meal for tea today.'

'I look pretty today.' etc

Every night read what you have written and keep these affirmations so you always have them to go back and re-read when you feel you need to.

Part two

Everyday I want you to really listen for compliments and positive things people say to you and again if you initially look for one and write it down. As you get more used to doing this you will hear more and more positives because you will be training yourself to now listen for the positives rather than the negatives. Like with part one every night read what you have written and let yourself believe it and accept it as true of you.

Part three

The last part is about you beginning to look after and nurture yourself. So once a week I want you to find some time for yourself and choose to do something lovely for yourself. Allow yourself at least one hour, more if you can, or you can build up to longer when you feel ready.

You may choose to have a long relaxing soak in the bath, or get a massage, or read a magazine or book, or watch a movie. It could be as simple as having an extra hour in bed it does not matter what you choose as long as it does not involve food and is something that benefits you and helps you feel better.

So we have to look past the food

Often by the time we realize we are using food in an unhealthy way, it feels like it has always been that way and we do not see an emotional link at all. We put it down to other things such as being big built, having a slow metabolism, too many fast food restaurants etc. Yet if we do take some time to just look back over our lives there will be an original pattern to our eating, even if now it just seems random.

If you stop and look back at the times you ate the most / least even when you were younger, or the times you were your heaviest / slimmest, you would probably be able to identify emotional issues going on at that time. Below is an exercise you can do that will further enable you to identify what part food has played throughout your life and give you more insight into the emotions you link to food.

Exercise

Get a pen and piece of paper and do a chart of significant events in your life from birth to the present and then underneath each event try to remember how you viewed and used food during those times and how that has shaped your eating patterns and your weight. Also think about the emotions you were feeling at those times and how these may have impacted your relationship with food.

Example

On my chart birthdays when I was a child would always be significant events, as I would have a party and sure enough they always revolved around food, even the games we played usually involved food because if you won the prize would often be sweets. For me emotionally birthdays were great as I was the centre of attention and got to feel special and the food was always food kids love like crisps, cake, sausage rolls etc, all the things we class as 'bad' foods.

It was a time I could eat anything I wanted. So for me

a lot of my happy times were linked to food and as mentioned earlier what can then happen is we associate these happy feelings with food rather than the event, the people etc. Subsequently as adults we try to recreate these feeling through food thinking the food will make us happy even though we know deep down it won't.

What really made me happy at my birthdays wasn't the food it was the whole event and the fact for that day I was special. So again we are back to feeling worthwhile about ourselves and the need to know we are valued and loved, which has nothing to do with food or what we eat.

Chapter 13

You cannot continue to blame, you must accept you have choices and control

While it can't be denied that fast food restaurants have shot up in numbers in the last thirty years and this without a doubt has had an impact upon our eating patterns, blaming the restaurants only serves to reinforce the illusion that you have no control over what you are doing and so you end up staying in your unhappy cycle with food, believing it is out of your control. If people had no control and no choice *everyone* would have unhealthy relationships with food and eat at fast food restaurants, which again is not the case.

People wonder how come very few people used to be obese, yet the reality is years ago food was not as readily available, there were no fast food restaurants, food did not have the additives in and there was not as much choice, so it would have been much harder to use food as an emotional crutch or get addicted to it.

Despite this though people will still have had emotional needs and ways of avoiding these needs just as they do today, the difference being they would not have been as able to use food as a means of trying to meet these needs or avoid their emotions.

We need to realize we are living in a 'blame' culture where people seem reluctant to acknowledge they have a choice but unless we accept we do, even if it's hard, we give up any power we have over our own lives and ultimately how *we* wish to live them. We end up unhappy blaming everything else and wondering why things don't change.

Making decisions can be hard but it is the only way we can reclaim power over our lives and our choices around our diet and make them how we want them to be. Fast food is not bad it can only be made bad by the way we choose to use it. Equally if you only ate salad every day, which is supposedly a 'good' food, you would not have a balanced diet and would end up ill. It is what **we choose** to do with food and how often **we decide** to eat it that makes it have a positive or negative effect on our lives and us. *This means that at the end of the day it is us that make the food become good or bad.*

Don't deny yourselves any foods, but maintain a balance

Having fast food as a treat every so often can actually be a 'healthy' thing to do because if we start thinking we cannot have a certain type of food what tends to happen is we crave that food and it can become an obsession. We think about it all the time and so eventually end up having it anyway, and then we feel bad because it was a food we were not 'supposed' to be having. Anyone who has smoked and then quit will know what I am talking about.

I remember when I was at university and trying to lose weight, I became obsessed, and I would look at cream cakes thinking, "Oh I can't have them even though they look so nice". I would have breakfast and straight away be thinking about what I could have for lunch because I thought I should not be eating between meals. So it became a real battle for me, and the funny thing was I didn't even like cream cakes, and I knew I couldn't be hungry straight after breakfast, but there was something about me believing I couldn't and shouldn't have cream cakes, eat between meals, etc. that made it the focus of a lot of my thinking. This in turn made it harder to resist doing.

What I needed to do was stop thinking about what I should or shouldn't have and learn to listen to my body and what it was telling me I needed, not what I thought I needed. What helped with this was I had a friend at university who had always been slim and what I noticed about her was she ate what she wanted yet never put on weight, and food was never an issue. Now I know you could say "well she was slim why would it be an issue?" but as you know that's not always the case, and equally, when in fact I became slim I was even more obsessed with food than when I was overweight because I was so frightened of putting the weight back on.

Anyway my friend, when she wanted a chocolate bar or felt hungry would just eat without the guilt, or thinking can I have this or I shouldn't have that, she was not worried about her weight. This really got me thinking about myself, and how I wished I could be like her in relation to food.

Slowly I began to realize that because my friend had a healthy relationship with food and it had no 'power' over her, she in turn was a healthy weight. She listened to her body and did not deprive herself of any food if she fancied it, so she never developed an unhealthy relationship with food, to her food was just food, which she enjoyed but it did not take over her life.

Learning to listen to our bodies is hard

Knowing this and putting it in to practice for me were two different things though, because I thought if I do just listen to and trust my body I will end up being overweight again, so although I was slim at the time I still viewed food in a negative way. As I have gotten older, and perhaps a little wiser, I am now able, like my friend, to eat what I want and stay the same weight. I have been a similar weight give or take a couple of pounds for over fifteen years now. I don't own any scales and I rarely get weighed. There is no point, I know by how I am eating and what's going on in my life emotionally if my relationship with food is beginning to get unhealthy, or the balance is slipping too much.

Subsequently I eat cakes, crisps, sweets, chocolate and go out for meals, but the difference is I now listen to my body and what it really needs, which often isn't food, it is something more, something that can't be filled or avoided by eating.

I am still aware I eat when I have emotional 'stuff' going on, or if I'm really stressed, but being aware of what I am doing enables me also to get the support I need, so the food does not take over and become tied in with what is going on for me emotionally.

For example I may have had a hard day at work and fancy something really nice to eat, which more often than not isn't a lettuce sandwich, so I have it. I don't feel guilty about it, I just allow myself to eat it while acknowledging why I am eating. This ensures I deal with the bigger issue of what is stressing me out at work and what I can do to restore the balance and feel alright again.

By taking responsibility you keep your power over your life

By looking at the bigger picture and taking responsibility I avoid using food as a crutch, I do not allow it to have any power over me. I maintain the power over my life. If you do not get the control back in your life and start taking responsibility for your actions, instead of blaming, you may never get what you need or find contentment. Eating for any other reason than hunger, unless done in awareness, will only lead to misery and further problems.

So as mentioned in chapter twelve you really need to think about what is missing in *your* life, what do *you* want out of your life, how can *you* get it and how can *you* start meeting your needs in an different more productive way. Only *you* can do this no one else.

As previously stated we cannot look to others for the answers, we can look to others for support but the answers to our questions can only be found in us. If we look hard enough, although it may be painful we will find them. What we find, and need to do might be hard but ultimately as adults *we* are responsible for our actions, and ourselves. If we are not happy in our life we need to reclaim our power back and look at what needs to change.

If we rely on others to make us happy we will be waiting forever because it is impossible for someone else to make you happy. People can add to your happiness and support you but they are not responsible for your life or your happiness, *you are*. Unfortunately, it is also not for me to say what is missing in your life, it is for you to find out and this may be a journey you are ready for and want to take or it may not. **Either way you are still ok, and need to learn to love and nurture yourself.**

Reading this book has started you on a journey, but only you can decide which path you take and where your journey leads you. One thing I can say for certain is if you do have an unhealthy relationship with food there will be something else going on emotionally that needs to be dealt with. It is up to you to decide whether or not you want to find out what the bigger picture is and deal with it. At the end of the day it is *your* life to choose to do what you want with, but remember every action and decision you make has a consequence that you ultimately have to live with.

Can you live with the consequences of your relationship with food?

The question to ask yourself is **"can you live with the long term consequences, of continuing with your unhealthy relationship with food?"** If you are reading this book the answer is no, because if you were happy as you are, or with your life, you would not be reading it.

Life is not always easy, but it can be great if we just let it. Life is full of ups and downs and we cannot escape this no matter how much we may want to. What we can do is make a choice as to how we deal with those ups and downs and how we look after ourselves in the most beneficial and healthy way. This will enable you to become more content in your life and feel better about yourself, which will ultimately have a positive impact on your relationship with food.

Chapter 14

An unhealthy relationship with food equals an unhealthy relationship with ourselves

We need to be clear that ultimately an unhealthy relationship with food is an unhealthy relationship with ourselves. If we really valued ourselves, our body and our health we would look after them.

Just because people look a certain way does not mean they have a 'good' relationship with food or themselves. People often assume that if we look how society wants us to (slim) we are healthy but this is a massive untruth, there are thousands of people who have problems with food, and their bodies, who look 'normal'. What is normal in our society unfortunately tends to be defined by the media and usually means being thin, which I for one don't agree with.

Having a healthy relationship with food and our bodies is not about being the perfect 10. Many people may be a size 10 but what they do to achieve this is far from healthy. We are all unique and we really need to start valuing this within ourselves, because in the end, deep down, we know whether or not we are looking after ourselves.

How can I fill my need?

By now you should be getting an idea of what is going on for you emotionally when you eat, what seems to be missing in your life or within you and / or what you are trying to avoid or fill with food. The million dollar question is how do you now get the need, or needs, you have identified met, so you no longer look to food for the solution.

The first step to any change is awareness because until something is in our awareness we have no ability to make a different choice, we have no choice. People without awareness often change for a while but then revert back to their old ways and this is also true with food, which is another reason why diets usually only work in the short term.

Becoming aware means we have a choice to do something different. Often this is not an easy choice because patterns of behaviour are hard to change especially long term but with awareness we can no longer avoid what we are doing.

For example if we have been eating to deal with our emotional issues but did not know this then how can we choose to change. However once we become aware this is what we are doing we now have the choice, we may choose not to change but the difference is *the choice is now there* whereas before it was not.

Frequently people with awareness will try to ignore what they know deep down because they don't want to be faced with a difficult choice and maybe have to deal with deep, painful emotional issues they have been trying to avoid for most of their lives. The real sadness in this is these people are actually often only existing or half living because they have limited their choices and therefore their lives.

This is often why people blame because it takes the focus off them, and while they are blaming they do not have to face the truth and take responsibility for their situation. For example when you ask people who are avoiding in this way what they eat, they will often distort the truth so they do not have to become aware.

So someone who eats for emotional reasons may on some level genuinely believe that they eat very little, or eat mainly healthy. They put their continued weight gain or health problems down to something else. They may even lie about what they have eaten while believing their lie to be true. I would bet if for one week they wrote down *everything* they ate they would be able to see the truth, but often this is too painful to face. The distortion allows them to stay the same believing they have no choice to be different.

What they fail to understand is when we do this nothing changes and we remain as we are, waiting for someone or something to make our lives better. Taking responsibility and accepting we have choices may seem hard but it gives us power over our lives. How amazing to realize we can make our lives how we want, *we can choose.*

How do I begin to get my needs met in a healthy way rather than through food?

Another way of looking at the question of how I can fill my need is; **"how do I begin to get my needs met in a healthy way rather than through food?"** I believe as a society we are very bad at meeting and recognizing our own needs because there is a myth that to do so is selfish, and we should always be putting others first. We learn to ignore what we need to be healthy and content and then wonder why we aren't. I am not condoning treating people in an unjust way or walking all over people to get what we want. What I am talking about is listening to our own bodies and minds and what they are telling us we require to stay healthy emotionally and physically. If we do not look after ourselves as adults who will?

When we are children it is the responsibility of our parents to meet our needs and look after us, but part of becoming an adult is the realization that we are now responsible for ourselves and have to get our own needs met, as *we are no longer dependants.*

This does not mean we cannot ask for support or let people do things for us but we have to understand they also have choices as adults and can choose to say no. We can then choose to ask someone else or meet the need ourselves. This is different from when we are children because as children we are dependant and rely on our parents for our survival.

For example a small baby if left alone for even a few hours would die because a baby cannot physically or emotionally meet any of its own needs; it is totally dependant on its carers for its survival and physical and emotional health. As we grow up this dependence gets less and less and we learn to look after ourselves and meet our own needs until we eventually become independent adults.

Adults therefore do not *require* anyone else to ensure they survive. We are more than capable of surviving on our own and looking after ourselves. So what I am saying is as adults we need to be able to know, recognize and ask for what we need, or meet our own needs because it is no longer the responsibility of someone else to do this.

I use the word 'need' instead of want because I think there is an important distinction between the two words. When I use the word need I am referring to something our bodies have to have to stay healthy emotionally and physically. For example we all need food and water to survive and companionship, shelter, medical care etc.

When we 'want' something we do not necessarily require it to remain healthy. For example I may want a glass of wine or a new pair of shoes, which is fine, but without them I will still survive. I am not saying we should not have wants because as discussed earlier everything is okay in moderation, what I am saying is our body if we let it will tell us what it really needs to stay healthy and balanced and this will not always be food.

We have to start really listening to our bodies

How many times have you really listened to your body's needs, not just in terms of food but also in terms of emotional needs? Humans are born very tuned in to their bodies they have to be to survive because initially we cannot communicate our needs verbally or meet them ourselves. As babies we are aware of when we are hungry, when we are wet, when we are tired, when we want attention, etc. and we make our needs known to our parents so they can meet them.

However, as we mature and become adults we seem to lose this instinctive connection to our bodies around how we are feeling and what we are needing, and despite being able to communicate and meet our own needs we don't. I believe this is because we have forgotten to tune in to ourselves and listen to what our bodies are telling us.

How do we begin to do this again so that we can become healthier happier individuals? How do we stop ignoring our needs or filling them with the wrong kinds of things like food, drink, drugs, sex, etc? The answer may appear a simple one but in reality after years of ignoring ourselves it is very hard to do, not only because we seem unable to listen to our needs but also even when we do we appear to have lost the ability to hear or recognize what our own bodies require.

This is why we end up filling our body full of food because it, or something else, becomes the substitute for what we really need, and what's even worse is we begin to believe that this substitute is what we really need, which is how we become addicted.

For a brief period the food makes us feel satisfied and appears to fill the need, but because it is not what our body is really craving it cannot possibly make us happy, content etc. As I have already said food can only work to fill a need if that need is physical hunger, you wouldn't try and repair a puncture with food would you? Yet we try and repair ourselves, and meet a lot of our needs through food, when it is totally unsuitable.

Just as repairing a puncture in an inappropriate way will only lead to more problems so will trying to make ourselves feel better through food. Initially it may fill the hole but quite soon afterwards the hole returns with even more force than before and requires something even bigger to fill it, so we eat more and so it continues.

Chapter 15

You need to stop and think before reaching for food

What we have to do is to start tuning in to our bodies, both emotionally and physically, so we can start to recognize what it is we really need at that time. Often when we are used to meeting a need through food it becomes automatic, we do it without thinking, so probably the first and most important step is to STOP AND THINK BEFORE YOU AUTOMATICALLY GO FOR FOOD.

This is where your food diary will help, because by doing it you will have seen how often you thought you were hungry, how often you were eating and what you were eating which should give you a sense of how much your food intake is actually down to hunger. For example if you found every hour or so you were eating then the reality is you are probably not hungry and there is something else going on.

How do you tell if it is hunger or not, and if not how do you identify what else it might be? A good starting point is to really stop and think before you just go for food. When you feel hungry sit with it for a while think about when you last ate, what you ate and how likely is it that your body should be hungry. Then ask yourself if I am not hungry what do I need?

Often when something has become a habit it is very difficult to break this pattern. The same is true for food, initially you may find it extremely hard to identify any other feeling but hunger because you are so used to associating all your feelings with being hungry, and trying to fill them this way. However if you persevere it will become easier and you will soon be re-tuning in to your body and what it actually requires.

So always stop before you eat and ask yourself the question; "is it logical that I am hungry bearing in mind when I last ate, and what I ate, or could there be something else going on?

Be aware of junk food as it does contain empty calories

An important thing to remember when thinking about this is that junk food does not fill you for long because it is not substantial, so what you often find is if you have eaten junk food for your meal you may feel hungry soon after.

The reality is still the same though that although you may feel hungry your body does not actually need food because you ate not long ago so you are not going to starve. This is why it is essential to have a balanced diet. Your body will crave foods that are substantial and fill its need for goodness, vitamins, minerals, etc. because that is how we survive and stay healthy.

We were not made to live on food full of fat, sugar, additives etc, as I'm sure you will already know. The point I am making is you are more likely to feel hungry if what you have been eating is all processed, sugar and takeaways. If this is true of you it would still suggest you have something else going on besides hunger, because if you valued yourself properly you would not be filling it all the time with foods that do not give your body what it really needs.

Again it goes back to listening to what our bodies need in order to be healthy, balanced and well, and the right diet plays a big part in that, as does our emotional health and getting our needs met enough of the time.

If you have a car and you want it to run smoothly and keep going and not get problems you look after it in certain ways. For most of the time the same is true of your body if you look after its needs it will be much more efficient and feel better and perform better than if you don't. This is not about denying ourselves things but about looking after ourselves and getting the balance right throughout our lives. Chances are if we can do this food would not be such a big issue anyway.

If you are not hungry what then?

So now you have stopped and thought about whether or not you are hungry, or more importantly, logically can you be hungry in terms of when you last ate, and what you ate, you now need to think about what else your body might need?

As I said earlier, initially you might struggle to get past the feeling that it's definitely hunger, and you may struggle to tune in to what else your body requires. This process of re-tuning into our bodies will not happen overnight, especially when a lot of us have been ignoring our own needs for so long, re-learning can take patience and time but the outcome should pay off.

The diary you kept will help by giving you an idea of what your needs might be when you feel you are hungry. You may find a theme emerges i.e. it always seems to be when I am stressed that I eat more, or when I feel bored, tired etc. The reality is it will probably be slightly different for everyone because we are all individuals, which is why there is no exact science, right answer, or magic wand that will make our relationship with food different.

Only we can make things different.

Most of it is about hard work from us and us choosing to take back the control and do something different. It is about us making the choice to invest in us, and life, **because we are worth it**, despite what we might have heard or have been told differently. We are all special, but often it is down to us to find that specialness within us and to hold onto it in a world where this is often difficult to do.

People may well say obesity never used to be a problem, so it's obviously down to people being lazy and fast food restaurants etc, and while the latter is true in terms of we do have more fast food restaurants and more processed food around than ever before, it is also true that *we* have a choice about where and what *we* eat. I agree that it is easier now than ever to have an unhealthy relationship with food but I would argue that for a lot of people if it wasn't food it would be something else, because it is about more than just food.

No one in their right frame of mind would want the problems obesity or anorexia bring, they may convince themselves everything is fine but that's only because the alternative feels too much for them to face.

People seem to have lost the ability in our society to take responsibility for their own actions and we seem to have given up wanting control over our lives, yet if we were to take this control back we can then make our lives how we want them to be. This may feel scary but again it goes back to being tuned in to your body and yourself, finding out what you want, what your needs are and being proactive in getting them met. Some people may need support to get there either from friends, family or professionals, and that's fine, because we are human and we all need relationships and support.

So how do you fill your need?

You start by going back to basics and listening to what your body's need is. Then you think about how you might begin to get this need met, what needs to change, what is missing, what will it take for you to invest in you and in your life, because at the end of the day it is *your* life and as an adult *you* are responsible for that life and the choices you make.

If your life is not how you want it to be ultimately it comes down to you to change it. Life is not always going to be easy but if you can get back to tuning in to you, knowing what you need and how to get this, and realizing you are **great** regardless, then although life may be hard at times, you will know what to do in order to keep yourself healthy emotionally and physically.

Conclusion

I think I have said enough now and have probably said a lot of what you already knew, *its time now for action* like the old saying 'actions speak louder than words.' You will not change things in your life just by reading this book, you have done the easy part the hard part is changing and maintaining the change but I know you have the strength within you to do whatever it takes. I BELIEVE IN YOU.

So I just want to say GOOD LUCK ON YOUR JOURNEY, I feel privileged to have played a small part in that journey and if you take nothing else from this book than the fact YOU ARE WORTHWHILE; I think that's fantastic.

About the Author

Tracy Hancock is a qualifed Psychotherapist, Counsellor and Social Worker, and has worked in the helping professions for fifteen years. She has also taught and supervised trainee counsellors and psychotherapists.

Her numerous qualifications include: an MA in Integrative Psychotherapy, Diploma in Integrative Psychotherapy, Diploma in Counselling and Diploma in Social Work.

Tracy has a great awareness of understanding and dealing with people's emotional issues, not only because of her training but also because of having had her own therapy for several years.

She has a passionate interest regarding weight issues, having herself been on a journey with her own relationship with food, which is where the idea for this book came from.

Tracy now has a good relationship with food and would like to share her knowledge of how to achieve this with others, so they to can change thier relationship with food into something positive.